Handbook of
Veterinary Clinical Research

Handbook of
Veterinary Clinical Research

Mark Holmes MA VetMB PhD MRCVS
Senior Lecturer in Preventive Veterinary Medicine
University of Cambridge

Peter Cockcroft MA MSc VetMB DCHP DipECBHM DVM&S MRCVS MILT
Cambridge Expert Vets
(Veterinary Education Training and Support)

Blackwell
Publishing

Blackwell Publishing editorial offices:
Blackwell Publishing Ltd, 9600 Garsington Road, Oxford OX4 2DQ, UK
   Tel: +44 (0)1865 776868
Blackwell Publishing Professional, 2121 State Avenue, Ames, Iowa 50014-8300, USA
   Tel: +1 515 292 0140
Blackwell Publishing Asia Pty Ltd, 550 Swanston Street, Carlton, Victoria 3053, Australia
   Tel: +61 (0)3 8359 1011

First published 2008 by Blackwell Publishing Ltd

ISBN: 978-1-4051-4551-0

Library of Congress Cataloging-in-Publication Data

Holmes, Mark A. (Mark Adrian), 1959–
    Handbook of veterinary clinical research / Mark Holmes, Peter Cockcroft.
        p. ; cm.
    Includes bibliographical references and index.
    ISBN-13: 978-1-4051-4551-0 (pbk. : alk. paper)
    ISBN-10: 1-4051-4551-X (pbk. : alk. paper)
    1. Veterinary medicine–Research–Methodology.   I. Cockcroft, Peter D.   II. Title.
    [DNLM: 1. Epidemiologic Methods–veterinary.   2. Research Design.   3. Veterinary Medicine.
    SF 780.9 H752h 2008]
    SF756.3.H36 2008
    636.089′550724–dc22

                         2007018852

A catalogue record for this title is available from the British Library

Set in 10/12pt Myriad
by Aptara Inc., New Delhi, India
Printed and bound in Singapore
by Utopia Press Pte Ltd

The publisher's policy is to use permanent paper from mills that operate a sustainable forestry policy, and which has been manufactured from pulp processed using acid-free and elementary chlorine-free practices. Furthermore, the publisher ensures that the text paper and cover board used have met acceptable environmental accreditation standards.

For further information on Blackwell Publishing, visit our website:
www.blackwellpublishing.com

For my family: Belinda, Henry, Miles, Isobel and Fleur (born 18/3/2007),
whose gestation coincided with that of this book (MAH)

For Elizabeth, Edward and Simon (PDC)

CONTENTS

PREFACE

There has been a recent trend within academia for the worth of veterinary clinical research to be undervalued. In the race to measure or quantify research output the impact factors of clinical journals and the financial income from clinical research grants have unfairly labelled this type of research as having a lesser importance. The absolute quality of research is independent of its subject; there is equal potential to conduct poor quality research at the forefront of high technology biomedical science as there is to conduct clinical research to the highest scientific paradigms within veterinary clinical practice.

The quality of research should be judged on the soundness of the methodology and the significance of the research question being asked. In order to provide the best possible care for the animals we treat we need to know the answers to questions about the diagnostic options and treatments available; in order to make informed decisions we need to have answers to questions about prognosis and outcomes. Clinical research using appropriate methodologies is the best way to provide the answers to these questions. It has a direct impact on the welfare of the animals under our care and it provides us and our colleagues with the information to optimize our decision-making.

The greatest amount of veterinary clinical work is performed in non-academic general or referral veterinary clinics and therefore the greatest information needs are generated here. These clinics are also presented with the most appropriate populations with which to answer these questions and so it is a logical conclusion that this is the best place to perform veterinary clinical research. A veterinary education prepares practitioners not only for clinical work but also provides many of the key skills and much of the scientific background knowledge that are required to perform clinical research. This book is designed to provide additional information and help readers extend their understanding of the concepts that are introduced in every veterinary curriculum, and ultimately help veterinarians increase the quantity and quality of veterinary clinical research, particularly that undertaken from within veterinary clinical practice.

The concept of this book led directly from the introduction of the Clinical Research Outreach Program (CROP) at the University of Cambridge, Department of Veterinary Medicine. The authors designed and introduced this short course and support structure under the umbrella of the Cambridge Infectious Diseases Consortium funded as part of the Veterinary Research Initiative financed by HEFCE and Defra. The course was set up in recognition of the vast untapped potential of veterinary practitioners to perform clinical research combined with the recognition of a considerable need for high quality clinical research to enable veterinary practice to be performed to current standards of evidence-based veterinary medicine. Having run this course for several years we continue to be surprised by the enthusiasm, hard work and dedication of clinicians involved in practice-based clinical research. We have also noted the way that conducting clinical research has proved to be a rewarding and intellectually stimulating activity for those practitioners who have embarked on this extension of their clinical activities.

We would like to thank our colleagues on the CROP course, particularly James Wood, Meg Staff, Fred Heath and Cerian Webb, who have contributed both directly and indirectly to the content of this book. Ian and Karen Mason provided valuable help on clarifying the legal issues covered in Chapter 16, however, any errors that may have crept in are entirely down to the authors' misinterpretation of their advice. One final acknowledgement is due to Stephen Hulley and his co-authors of *Designing Clinical Research*, published by Lippincott Williams & Wilkins and now in its third edition. Much of the structure and content of our handbook has been inspired by their work, which we have used as a textbook on the CROP course since its inception.

Mark Holmes
Peter Cockcroft
Cambridge, 23rd March 2007

INTRODUCTION

What is the best way to introduce a book on veterinary clinical research? Almost everything in this introductory chapter alludes to the bedrock of clinical research, so the first request is for readers not to skip this chapter as 'probably of general interest only'. The use of quotations may be perceived as an affectation used by authors to suggest to their readers a greater level of wisdom (or possibly education) than the author's own words convey. However, the following two quotations summarize all that follows.

> 'I know nothing except the fact of my ignorance.'
> Socrates quoted by Diogenes Laertius in *Lives of the Philosophers*

> 'If I have seen further it is by standing on the shoulders of giants.'
> Isaac Newton, in a letter to Robert Hooke, 5 February 1676

So, acknowledge your ignorance, look for giants, and read on.

1.1   What is veterinary clinical research?

There are a variety of possible definitions for the term 'veterinary clinical research' but most of them will include a reference to patients or the direct applicability of the results to the veterinary diagnosis, treatment or prognosis of disease in animals. Clinical research is often thought of as 'applied' research, as if this might distinguish it from other forms of more pure research. The word 'science' is rarely mentioned and yet good clinical research is nothing more or less than scientific research. Clinical research is performed because whatever our motivations we all share a desire to learn the 'truth' or at least take a step towards something we can have some confidence is more representative of the truth than the knowledge we had before.

We live in an age in which there is tremendous confusion between science and technology.

While developments in technology are dependent on scientific progress and these developments speed up the advance of science, science and technology are not synonymous. Science is a method that is designed to seek knowledge (i.e. truth); technology is the mere application of that knowledge.

One cannot fail to be impressed (and occasionally dismayed) at the ingenuity of technologists. Our mechanical engineers, computer scientists and applied geneticists, for example, astound the world with ingenuity and endeavour. However, without wishing to belittle their contribution, the modern motor car, the personal computer and genetically modified plants are constructed so that they *will* work, based on the knowledge that has been produced by science. The designers of complex electronic devices cleverly integrate hundreds or thousands of components that have already been shown to work in isolation and develop new devices that are faster and more sophisticated but the designers do not wire up all the components of a consumer electronic device to ask the question 'Will it work?'

Clinical research is just an area of scientific research. Like laboratory-based research it can be done well and it can be done badly; it is performed by people who share the same human frailties as the rest of humankind. Clinical scientists have the same hopes and fears of success and failure as everyone else, and they will make mistakes and errors of judgement. The preferred tool they have to guide them in their attempts to progress along the path to 'truth' is the strict adherence to a systematic methodological approach called the 'scientific method'.

1.2   What is the 'scientific method'?

We take it for granted, as a result of our education, that the Earth and other planets orbit the Sun and that the passage of day and night is a result of the Earth's rotation, but stop for a moment and imagine what it must have been like some 4000 years ago. Why would you think that you and the ground beneath your feet were moving at thousands of miles an hour? Why wouldn't you think that the Sun was moving across the sky above a stationary Earth? Ptolemy, among others, propounded this geocentric view of the universe and Eudoxus came up with an explanation of why different celestial objects move at different speeds: each set is embedded within concentric crystal spheres (rotating at different speeds) with the Earth in the centre (see Fig. 1.1). There was one sphere for the Sun, one for the Moon, one for the stars and one each for the planets. This model worked fairly well other than the slightly odd behaviour of the planets. The very name of these celestial bodies suggests the problem; the word planet is derived from a word meaning 'the wanderers'. These planets had the annoying habit of occasionally moving backwards for a period before resuming their normal movement.

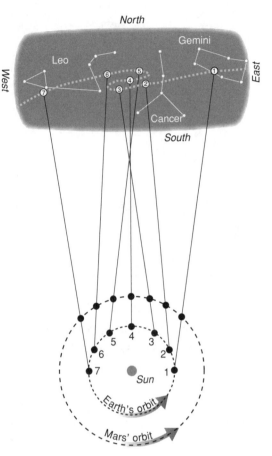

Figure 1.2 Diagrammatic representation of the apparent retrograde motion of Mars against the backdrop of the stars.

With our 'correct' knowledge we realize that the appearance of backward motion results from the fact that the Earth is orbiting the Sun and we are observing another object in a solar orbit (see Fig. 1.2). This retrograde movement didn't really fit the constantly spinning spheres idea. The Ptolemaic solution was to introduce a circle on the surface of the sphere that spun round and thus accounted for this aberrant retrograde motion (Fig. 1.3). Several thousand years later a Polish priest called Nicolaus Copernicus began to realize that a much simpler explanation for the movement of the planets might be a heliocentric model of the universe, placing the Sun in the

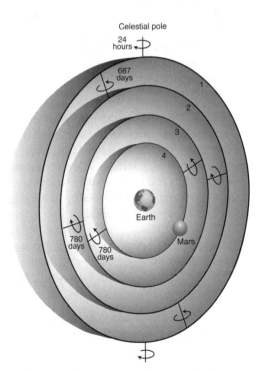

Figure 1.1 Illustration of the celestial spheres model of the universe described by Eudoxus.

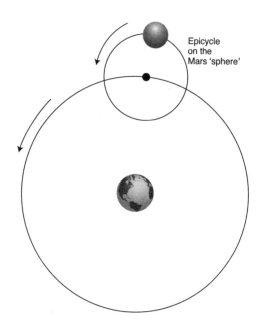

Figure 1.3 The Ptolemeic explanation of retrograde motion using an epicycle on the orbit of Mars.

middle, with the Earth spinning and the other planets also orbiting the Sun. This could also account for other phenomena such as the seasons if the Earth was tilted on its axis. His work paved the way for Galileo, Keppler, Brahe and others who, using this model, began to make better predictions about the behaviour of celestial bodies. These predictions were made with increasing accuracy, and as the evidence supporting a heliocentric model increased, it became increasingly difficult to dismiss the possibility of this new view of the universe.

We take the scientific knowledge we possess now for granted but what we should ask ourselves is why we believe this knowledge to be true.

The contemporary educational approach in the UK is to introduce science by encouraging children to make predictions based on prior observations. The sort of exercise that might be used would be to ask 'What do snails eat?' The children might suggest lettuce, grass, dead leaves or

cheese. The teacher might put all these potential feedstuffs into a vivarium with some snails and ask the children what they predict will happen. Hopefully one of the children will predict that the lettuce will disappear as it gets eaten, and if the teacher is lucky the snails will engorge themselves on the lettuce. In this way the children are introduced to observation, generating a hypothesis and testing, the keystones of science.

One of the key elements of scientific method is the concept of 'falsifiability' expounded by the philosopher Karl Popper in the 1920s. Popper believed that no empirical hypothesis, proposition or theory can be considered scientific if it does not admit the possibility of a contrary case or a contradicting observation: a hypothesis that all swans are white could be proved wrong by the simple test of seeing a black swan. This has two consequences: the first is that if a test cannot be performed (or envisaged) then it is not scientific, the second is that we can never achieve a scientific certainty – we can only state that the hypothesis has not failed any tests performed so far. By employing scientific method we may not be able to see into the future but we can have some confidence in the observations we have made in the past.

A clinical example that might make you think is a very personal story from a distinguished medical practitioner and researcher. Iain Chalmers bought a copy of Dr Benjamin Spock's famous book *Baby and Child Care* when he was a recent medical graduate in the mid-1960s. In his copy he marked a passage that read:

> 'There are two disadvantages to a baby's sleeping on his back. If he vomits, he's more likely to choke on the vomitus. Also he tends to keep his head turned towards the same side . . .
>
> . . . I think it is preferable to accustom a baby to sleeping on his stomach from the start.'

As an obstetrician Iain Chalmers passed on and acted on this apparently rational and authoritative advice in Dr Spock's book. Collation of the results of many simple observational

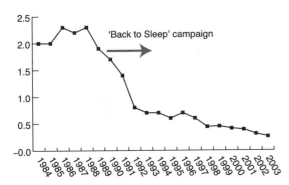

Figure 1.4 The effect on infant mortality (deaths per thousand births) of the 'Back to Sleep' health campaign launched in the late 1980s.

studies contradicted this advice and culminated in the launch of a public health campaign in the late 1980s ('Back to Sleep'), recommending that infants should be placed on their backs to sleep in order to reduce the risk of sudden infant death syndrome (SIDS). As a result of this campaign the rate of deaths attributed to SIDS was reduced from about 2 per 1000 births to about 0.5 per 1000 births (Blair et al., 2006; Fig. 1.4). In a letter to the *British Medical Journal* Iain Chalmers wrote 'We now know that the advice promulgated so successfully in Spock's book led to thousands, if not tens of thousands, of avoidable cot deaths' (Chalmers, 2001). This should be a sobering warning to those of us who disseminate or apply health information without ensuring, to the best of our ability, that evidence from reliable empirical research has shown that our prescriptions and proscriptions are more likely to help than to harm our patients.

While this example supports the use of good quality clinical research and effective communication, it also illustrates the fundamental scientific principles that underpin the practice of veterinary medicine as applied by an individual practitioner caring for an individual patient. Of course there are important skill sets other than an ability to critically appraise the scientific literature that contribute to our performance as veterinarians. A good clinician needs good powers of observation, an empathy with both patients and clients, manual dexterity, and a host of other skills. But apart from these we need to accept that our clinical decisions might be wrong and to constantly ask the question 'Can I obtain better information that can reduce this uncertainty?'

1.3 Errors and truth

To lay out a grand ambition, the goal of humankind is to learn the truths of the universe. While philosophers and theists can ponder the limitations of the empirical approach, scientists perform experiments in order to make observations; an experiment is really just a convenient arrangement to make observation possible. From the observations made the scientist makes an inference, i.e. an assumption that what is observed has a more general applicability.

The goal of the clinical researcher is to infer from the results of a clinical study the truth as it applies to their research question (Fig. 1.5). The first step is to formulate the research question, the second step is to design the study or experiment, and the third step is to perform the study. Having obtained the results from the study an inference is made that the results reflect the truth that was present in the study population and then infer that the truth in the study population reflects a more general truth (Fig. 1.6).

There are four main areas where fundamental errors can be introduced: the study design, the study implementation, incorrect inferences from the actual results and incorrect inferences from the study to the wider population.

The first error may be caused by designing a study that doesn't actually answer the question we are asking. Even if the study design addresses the question it may fail to be implemented according to the research protocol. Once the results are obtained errors in the analysis of the results may fail to identify the truth in the study population. While this may be due to human error (a systematic error), it may also be due to chance (randomness). The final area for error is

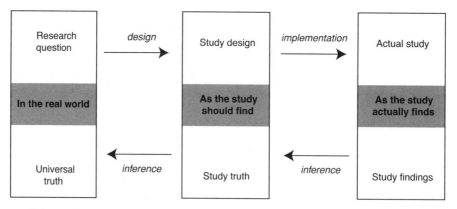

Figure 1.5 Schematic representation of the relationship between clinical research and the 'truth' in the real world.

in the incorrect inference from the study results to the broader population, which may be due to a systematic error (i.e. the study population or situation does not reflect the 'whole world') or again may be due to chance (e.g. by luck the animals that were selected were unrepresentative of the broader population).

From this discussion it can be seen that there are two areas from which errors can be generated: from our design and implementation of the study or by chance. A good knowledge of the subject area, methodical rational reasoning and an adherence to the best clinical research practices should reduce the likelihood of systematic errors occurring. Errors due to chance can be minimized by the appropriate use of statistics both during the design of research studies and in the analysis of results.

1.4   Why do we perform veterinary clinical research?

Few people would contradict the assertion that the goal of scientific researchers is to discover the 'truth' or at least to provide evidence in support of a particular 'truth'. However, it would be naïve

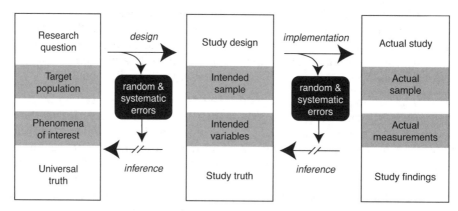

Figure 1.6 Schematic representation of the process of clinical research and where errors can affect inferences about the 'truth'.

to believe that this search for truth is the only motivation for the vast majority of researchers. Depending on our circumstances we are likely to be motivated by the perception of our work by our peers, the need to have work published as a prerequisite for a qualification, the need to accumulate a body of scientific publications for career advancement, or the need for publications to attract further funding for our research work. The danger in this is that the publication becomes more important than the research. Of course, publication is an essential part of the process; there is little point in performing research and failing to communicate the results but if we measure our performance according to the quantity of the research performed rather than the quality of the research it is tempting to lower our standards.

The personality of the researcher may introduce a further bias. The enemy of good research is dogma or a closed mind. Where a researcher has established a reputation on a particular body of work, leading to a widespread belief in a particular model or theory, it may become difficult for that researcher to accept evidence that challenges this accepted belief. Very few researchers embark on a study without anticipating a particular result and it is easy for expectation to manifest itself as a desire for that result. While it is appropriate to question an unexpected result, review our methodology and even to repeat the experiment, very few of us subject our expected result to the same level of scepticism or doubt.

Hope, fear and desire are human characteristics that make it hard for us to make accurate judgements about risk; however, these same characteristics also impede our objectivity when performing clinical studies. We can protect our research from *ourselves* by techniques such as randomization and blinding in our study designs but it is important to be self-aware about our human weaknesses in every aspect of our research work. When we read the literature, review other people's papers and grants, and when we write up our own studies we should strive to be objective. The most valuable tool in our intellectual armoury is an open mind. Genuine constructive scepticism is part of having an open mind, i.e. we are able to entertain the possibility of an alternative explanation for what has been stated or suggested. The open mind does not mean an empty mind; an empty open mind would never manage to reach a conclusion. A good breadth and depth of background knowledge is essential. Veterinarians are fortunate in that we receive good training in a wide variety of biological disciplines. Effective clinical research requires a thorough knowledge of literature in the research area and in this way judgements can be made from a platform of knowledge (appraised evidence).

1.5 Research from practice

In a letter to *The Veterinary Record* (16 September 2006), a veterinary practitioner noted that only 6% of the papers in the main veterinary clinical journals were written by practitioners, while 96% of practitioners would like to read papers written by their fellow practitioners. There is little doubt that practitioners are an underutilized source of knowledge and potential research. There is a strong feeling among practitioners that it is difficult to get papers published in peer-reviewed veterinary journals, and they are often disheartened by the responses from the reviewers of their papers.

While some of the conventions of scientific writing may seem arbitrary (e.g. the use of the passive third person tense) the systematic conduct of scientific investigations and the clear communication of all elements of a study are very important. Although it might seem unfair to subject practitioners' research to the same degree of scrutiny as research performed by full-time veterinary researchers, the nature of truth is absolute and the consequences of promulgating incorrect information may be grave.

While excellent research continues to be undertaken and published by practitioners, the majority of research emanating from university departments and research institutes is conducted by investigators who have undertaken formal research training. Just as a new graduate might not be expected to undertake complex orthopaedic surgery, there are research skills and specialized knowledge that help investigators to conduct studies and improve the quality of the subsequent communication of their results. While such training can certainly not guarantee the value of the research performed, or the conclusions drawn from it, it can help to reduce the barriers that prevent the publication of more practice-based research.

Training can be acquired from self-education by reading books such as this one, from part-time or distance learning courses (details of the Cambridge Clinical Research Outreach Program can be found at http://www.vet.cam.ac.uk/cidc/training/outreach.html), and through working with a more experienced colleague or mentor. Formal training is a good place to start but the best learning experience is acquired through performing research. Much practical advice is provided in the following chapters but the best advice that can be given to a practitioner embarking on a project for the first time is not to do it alone. While not every academic

will be able or willing to provide supervision or be your mentor, you will be surprised to learn that there is an enormous amount of goodwill towards practitioners and a willingness to collaborate with practice-based colleagues. If you are unsure who to contact then a good place to start would be the authors of papers written describing clinical research in your field of interest. The first academic or researcher you approach may not necessarily respond but if you are persistent you are likely to find someone who is willing to help. Bear in mind that if you don't ask they can't say 'yes' or 'no'. Don't despair if the partnership doesn't work out; like any relationship, the relationship between an investigator and their mentor, supervisor or collaborator may break down or never really flourish. All relationships require work and often break down only as a result of poor communication.

1.6   References

Blair PS, Sidebotham P, Berry PJ, Evans M, Fleming PJ (2006) Major epidemiological changes in sudden infant death syndrome: a 20-year population-based study in the UK. *Lancet* Jan 28 **367** (9507): 314–19.

Chalmers I (2001) Invalid health information is potentially lethal [letter]. *BMJ* **322**: 998.

2

ESTABLISHING THE HYPOTHESIS

Objectives

After reading this chapter readers should:

- be able to identify the characteristics of a good research question
- be able to translate research questions into formal hypotheses
- understand the statistical principles underlying the testing of a hypothesis.

2.1   What is the question?

As has already been implied, good clinical research concentrates on a single focused research question. At each stage of the study we should be asking or reminding ourselves of the question that we are trying to answer. We will get distracted by the opportunities to ask additional secondary questions, opportunities to collect ancillary data and by the practical problems of conducting our research. The study should be justified by the strength or value of our primary question. A poor research question is not redeemed because our study design enables us to answer several other questions or collect extra information.

What makes a good question in clinical research? The best clinical research addresses a question that has arisen in the clinic. The results generated from a good clinical research question influence a decision made during the diagnosis or treatment of a patient. In other words a veterinarian (somewhere at some time) wants or needs the answer to our question in order to provide the best care for a patient.

We also have to be realistic about our motivation and our goals. A pharmaceutical company is ultimately motivated by profits and has greater resources than an academic clinician looking to advance their career during post-graduate training. We need to be aware of our potential for subjectivity and our potential to introduce unintentional bias; adherence to the principles of scientific method will help to ensure the integrity of the results of our research.

2.2   What are the characteristics of a good research question?

A good research question should be feasible, interesting, novel (ideally but not essentially), ethical and relevant.

2.2.1   Feasibility

There are many practical reasons why the question we want to ask may not be feasible. This may lead us to narrow our focus or modify our question. It is far better to successfully answer a more limited question than it is to get 75% through a larger study and fail to answer the question.

Number of patients/subjects

Many studies falter due to over-optimistic estimates of the number of cases that can be enrolled. Many clinical researchers believe that there is a malevolent force in the universe that reduces the incidence of even the most common conditions once they start recruiting cases of that disease. The first and most important step is to conduct a sample size estimate (see Chapter 6). The more prior data we have the better this estimate will be. In essence we need to know what we are going to measure, how much it is likely to vary (an estimate of the variance) and what magnitude of effect we would like to be able to detect. This is to avoid the problem of failing to have sufficient statistical power in our study to demonstrate a statistically significant effect. Once we know how many cases we need then we should be able to establish if it is feasible to recruit or enrol the cases needed. Firstly we can use the historical case records from our own clinic for an incidence estimate. How long will it take to complete the study? What are our inclusion criteria? How many cases will be lost through exclusion criteria? How many clients are likely to decline to participate? How many will be lost to follow-up? All these questions need to be considered. A pilot study may be worth considering to provide more accurate values for these parameters.

When numbers or the rate of recruitment look poor then it may be worth looking to involve collaborators or other clinics, widening the inclusion criteria, reducing unnecessary exclusions, extending the duration of the study and ultimately considering using a different study design. The quality of evidence from a retrospective case-control study may be less good than a randomized controlled trial but when cases are thin on the ground it may be our only option.

Technical feasibility

Consider carefully the skills, equipment and experience that will be needed to perform the study. Apart from the purely veterinary expertise and hardware that will be required there are the logistical problems of collecting and analysing the data. The best strategy will be to use familiar and established approaches to reduce the uncertainty of developing new skills and procedures. If there are obvious gaps in your own expertise it is advisable to recruit a collaborator to be involved from the beginning of the planning process. In particular it is often wise to include a statistician or epidemiologist in the research team.

Financial and time costs

While much clinical research can be performed with very little money it is important not to underestimate the time and effort that may be required. If the study plan requires busy clinicians to complete extensive additional paperwork during the course of their normal veterinary work we may find that initial goodwill will rapidly disappear. Be practical and realistic in the demands that are made on participants. How much data is really essential to answer the project question? If this is your first clinical research project err on the side of caution and keep things simple. Again a short pilot phase is enormously helpful in establishing just how much work is really involved. We need to ensure that the quality of work performed at the tail end of the study is just as good as that at the start.

2.2.2 Interest

The greatest difficulty that many veterinarians have when embarking on clinical research is to find an answerable question that holds their interest. This difficulty arises out of the breadth of vision that we have and the complexity of the clinical process that is involved in animal health care. Somehow simple research projects seem too trivial but the study design required to answer the question we'd really like to ask is too broad in scope. Just as we wouldn't expect a new graduate to embark on complex orthopaedic reconstructions we need to acknowledge our own inexperience in research methodology and relevant clinical research experience. Try to find a focused question related to the 'big' question. There is almost no point in conducting research in a subject area that holds no interest as it will never be conducted with rigor and discipline, but we have to match our goals to our abilities. The big question can be answered piece-by-piece but maybe not in one heroic study.

2.2.3 Novelty

The need for novelty is always emphasized by the research funding bodies and the publishers of scientific papers but this makes the frightening assumption that researchers never get things wrong. No clinical researcher would be particularly interested in repeating something that was well-established by the results of previous research; however, there are plenty of examples of studies involving small numbers of animals or studies using flawed methodology that need to be repeated before we can be certain of their findings. There should be a clear rationale for clinical research that is not novel. Veterinarians who disagree with the opinions of the veterinary establishment should not hesitate to perform a critique of the relevant literature and test these opinions by either repeating existing studies or conducting studies with better designs to provide evidence to either confirm or refute the existing dogma. In the human field clinical trials and epidemiological studies are frequently repeated and subsequently analysed collectively to improve the quality of the overall finding. While it may be many years before meta-analyses are common in the veterinary literature, there is clearly some value in repeating existing studies in new populations.

2.2.4   Ethical issues

Within the UK there are clear legal issues that need to be addressed to avoid falling foul of data protection legislation and to ensure that studies do not fall under the scope of the Animal (Scientific Procedures) Act 1986. Beyond this there are also issues surrounding the informed consent of clients. If there is any doubt then an independent ethical opinion should be sought (see Chapter 16).

2.2.5   Relevance

When we appraise the veterinary literature we first determine if the results are likely to be true (an appraisal of the methodology employed and the statistical analysis) and if the results are important (do we care about them). Firstly, there is the magnitude of the effect reported: a difference in the success of a treatment may be reported to be statistically significant but be so slight as to be useless (this can happen when a large number of animals are included in a trial). Secondly, is this research about a condition or situation that we are likely to encounter? Ideally veterinary clinical research should be designed to provide an answer that would be relevant to a veterinarian in general practice and not just to a highly specialized practitioner in an exceptionally well-equipped veterinary hospital. Researchers should be guided by their own judgement and opinion but if the opportunity arises to broaden the relevance to a wider population of animals with little extra effort the results may be applied to provide a greater good.

2.3   Selecting the research questions

The primary question should be carefully selected, clearly defined and stated from the outset.

The question must be answerable (i.e. feasible, as discussed above) and will provide our hypothesis (described below); however, in the design of the study there will be a number of further aspects of our research question that need consideration.

2.3.1   Secondary questions

With almost any research the study design will lend itself to providing answers to other questions. These secondary questions should not be allowed to compromise the study's ability to answer the primary question. The study may be designed from the outset to answer these additional questions (taking the opportunity to collect extra data) or the data collected for the primary question may also provide data for ancillary questions.

The secondary questions may be of two types. In the first type the secondary question uses different outcome variables. In a drug trial the primary question may look at the efficacy of two treatments while secondary questions may measure the incidence of adverse effects. In the second type of question the same outcome variable is used but the analysis uses different subgroups for analysis. Secondary questions about sex or breed influence on the outcome are an example of this type of question.

It is important that any subgroups that are going to be used to address secondary questions are:

- specified at the design stage
- chosen on a rational basis (i.e. with reasonable expectations)
- limited in number.

As the numbers within the subgroups are not under the investigator's control, numbers may well be too small to establish a statistically significant result. These secondary questions may still be of value as hypothesis generators.

2.3.2   Adverse effects

Measurement of some adverse effects can be predicted from prior knowledge. For example, a trial comparing cyclosporine to prednisolone for the treatment of canine atopic dermatitis (Olivry et al., 2002) anticipated adverse effects on the gastro-intestinal system associated with cyclosporine and polyuria/polydipsia associated with prednisolone. Other adverse effects may be impossible to anticipate. Serious pharmacological toxicity should have been eliminated prior to clinical trials and will be highly unlikely in drugs that have been licensed. Nonetheless a health monitoring protocol, client education and clear routes for communication are an important aspect of study design where adverse effects may be anticipated.

2.4   The hypothesis

If the research question does not translate quickly and easily into a testable hypothesis then it is likely that a good research question hasn't been chosen. The main significance of establishing the hypothesis is that it will dictate the approach used for statistical analysis; however, it is worth attempting to formulate a formal hypothesis at an early stage as it may reveal the likely problems in designing a scientifically rigorous study that is able to answer the question. There is always a 'chicken and egg' element here (i.e. which comes first, the study design or the formal hypothesis) but even if the hypothesis changes when the study design is finalized it is still extremely valuable to lay one out at an early stage.

The hypothesis is a careful rewording of the question in the form of the expected result and precisely defines what the study is designed to test.

If the question is 'Is drug X an effective treatment for condition feline hyperthyroidism?' then the hypothesis might be 'Treatment of cats suffering from hyperthyroidism with X reduces the levels of thyroid hormone measured from blood samples taken 7 days after the start of treatment compared with samples taken prior to treatment.' In statistical terms this is called (somewhat confusingly) the 'alternative hypothesis' because the statistical tests will be used to reject the 'null hypothesis'. The null hypothesis is that 'There is no difference in the levels of thyroid hormone measured from blood samples taken 7 days after the start of treatment compared with samples taken prior to treatment in cats treated with X suffering from hyperthyroidism.'

Stating the research question as a hypothesis at an early planning stage is a good way of establishing the focus of the question. A clear definition of each term in the hypothesis is required. Referring to the example above: What do we mean by 'cats'? What is the population to be sampled? What is the case definition for 'hyperthyroidism'? How are the 'thyroid levels' going to be measured? How is the blood sample to be taken (are we using whole blood, serum or plasma)? When we say 'reduced', what level of reduction would be clinically useful? Why did we choose 7 days as the time period?

In general, the more precision and greater detail we can put into our hypothesis the easier the planning becomes as this reflects the decisions that have been taken to focus the question. On the other hand, this needs to be balanced against making unnecessarily proscriptive decisions at a stage when insufficient information is available. At the end of the planning process the hypothesis should be re-examined and amended (if necessary) to reflect the actual study design to be used. It is also worth asking if the hypothesis that is being tested still reflects the question that the investigator originally wished to address.

If the hypothesis is that there is no difference (e.g. a drug to be tested is as good as an existing treatment) then this indicates that the study is what is called an 'equivalence study' and there are some statistical ramifications that will need to be addressed (see Chapter 5).

2.5   The question doesn't translate into a hypothesis

A vague question will not translate into a simple hypothesis, and the first question the investigator should ask themselves is 'Can the research question be refined to help with the identification of a testable hypothesis?'

Although good science always asks simple focused questions, not all questions generate a hypothesis. Some questions ask a purely descriptive question such as 'What is the prevalence of West Nile Virus seropositive horses in the UK?' When there is no pre-existing data in the literature this is a valuable and useful subject for research and is often used to generate hypotheses for further research and provide baseline data. The important issues in the study design that will need attention are the population sampling method and establishing a sample size that will produce appropriate confidence limits for the result.

These types of studies are often surveys that collect additional information to allow subgroup analysis with subsequent multiple post-hoc analyses. They are relatively easy to perform but they are notoriously difficult to do well. If they are driven by an underlying question or idea such as 'The import of horses from the USA has caused some concern that West Nile Virus may have been introduced into the UK', it may be better to design a study that is hypothesis driven by comparing a cohort of imported horses from the USA with a control cohort (i.e. a group of horses matched by current location or a group imported from another source). The simpler focused question will produce a fairly unequivocal result assuming the study is properly designed, while a broader survey with multiple secondary questions has considerable potential to produce equivocal and misleading results.

2.6   Initial study design

Research design is an iterative process and although a good question may generate a testable hypothesis, problems may only become evident once the practicalities of study design are considered. A schematic representation of the process is provided in Fig. 2.1.

At an early stage the investigator should put his or her initial thoughts down on a one- or two-page project outline. This outline should begin to address the elements shown in Table 2.1. As confidence in the research question and hypothesis are established, the practical considerations of the study design needed to test the hypothesis need to be addressed. At the project outline stage it is likely that a putative study design type will be identified (e.g. case-control study, cohort study, randomized controlled trial, etc.); these are described in the following chapters. Answers to other questions such as 'How will the patients be selected?', 'What measurements will be taken?' and 'How many patients will be needed?' may not be answered but strategies to obtain the information to provide answers to these questions can be established.

2.6.1   Selecting a study design

A variety of study design types are described in some detail in the following chapters. In many instances the study type will be dictated by the animals or the clinical material available to the investigator; however, it is important to realise that the evidence generated from some study types provide stronger evidence than that generated from other study types. As the goal of clinical research is to provide good evidence on which our fellow veterinarians can base their clinical decisions it behoves us to choose a study design that will produce the strongest evidence possible.

The hierarchy of evidence (see Fig. 2.2) is a broad categorisation of study types highlighting those that are the most likely to produce the best evidence. In most clinical situations the value of

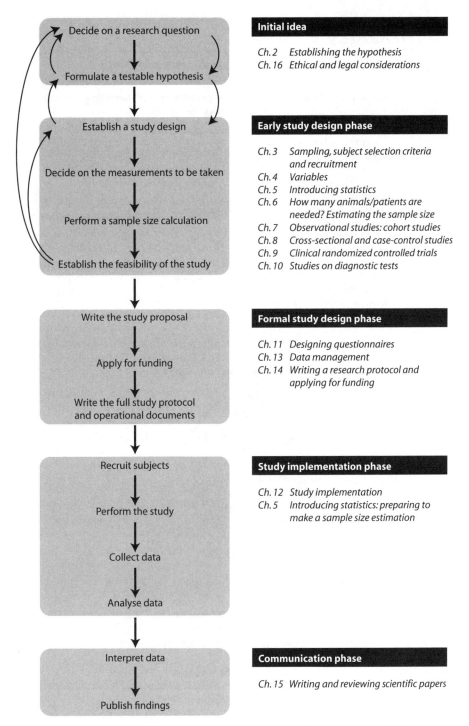

Figure 2.1 Diagrammatic representation of the tasks involved in veterinary clinical research, indicating sources of information in this book.

Table 2.1   Elements of the veterinary clinical research proposal.

Element	Questions
Research question	What questions will the study address? What is the principal hypothesis to be tested?
Background (significance)	Why should the research be performed? Why is it important?

Design
  Time frame for the study
  Study design type
	How is the study structured?

Subjects
  Selection criteria
  Sampling strategy
	Who are the subjects, what population will they come from and how will they be selected?

Variables
  Predictor variables
  Confounding variables
  Outcome variables
	What measurements will be taken?

Statistical issues
  Hypothesis
  Sample size
  Analysis (statistical tests)
	How many subjects will be required and how will the data be analysed?

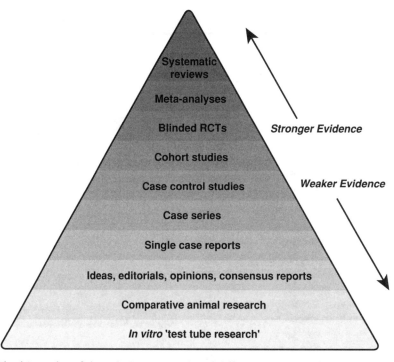

Figure 2.2 The hierarchy of the relative strengths of different sources of published evidence illustrated as a pyramid of evidence.

Table 2.2 The research question and study design: problems and solutions.

Potential problem	Solutions
Research question is too vague	Revisit the research question – can it be refined? Decide on a research question at an early stage Be specific in the early study plan and address the questions: 　Which population will subjects be drawn from? 　How will the subjects be sampled? 　How will the variables be measured?
Research question is too broad to be feasible	Specify a smaller set of variables Narrow the question
Too few subjects available	Expand the inclusion criteria Reduce the exclusion criteria Expand the sources of patients Lengthen the time frame of the study Consider strategies to decrease the required sample size (Chapter 6)
The skills of the investigator are limiting	Collaborate with colleagues who have the necessary skills Consider the use of alternative methodology Acquire the necessary skills
Study is too expensive	Consider other sources of funding Consider less costly study designs, e.g. fewer subjects and measurements, less extensive measurements, fewer follow-up visits
Research question is not interesting, novel or relevant	Consult with mentor/supervisor Reconsider the need for novelty Modify the research question
Research question has uncertain ethical acceptability	Consult with ethical review board Consider modifying the research question Consider the use of alternative methodology

evidence is directly proportional to the statistical power of the study. The power of the study indicates the ability of the study to demonstrate a difference. The power of a study is dependent on the size of the study population, the magnitude of the effect of the intervention, and the natural variation in the parameters being measured.

The greatest statistical certainty comes from well conducted meta-analyses (see Chapter 17) that incorporate a number of randomised controlled experimental studies (see Chapter 9). Because of the large number of participants the results are more reflective of the population as a whole. Similarly systematic reviews also provide strong evidence (also described in Chapter 17).

The randomised control trial (RCT) will ordinarily have the greatest power when compared to other data collection designs but it may not be appropriate to answer questions about causation where cohorts (Chapter 7) or case control (Chapter 8) studies are more appropriate. Randomised controlled trials are the design of choice for evidence regarding treatments. Trial designs further down the pyramid produce results that are less transferable to other populations but may be more applicable to certain types of patient. The object of the evidence hierarchy is to indicate the study design types most likely to yield the greatest rewards.

While individual case reports represent relatively poor evidence they may be extremely helpful in the absence of any other information and provide an appropriate way of describing the first occurrence of a new disease or clinical phenomenon. There is also overlap between the different levels in the hierarchy since a well-designed cohort study, may provide better evidence than a poorly designed RCT.

2.7   Problems with the research question and study design

A list of the potential problems and some possible solutions are given in Table 2.2. When considerable efforts have been expended, possibly with the acquisition of pilot data, it is tempting to soldier on and try to ignore substantial flaws as it may be assumed that these flaws cannot be addressed without starting again from scratch. Resist the urge to just carry on and seek advice if this should happen. Sharing the problem with others and seeking advice will often reveal a solution. The value in having a mentor or supervisor for the project or having recruited other members of the research team will become evident when this happens (and will often prevent problems at a much earlier stage).

2.8   Reference

Olivry T, Steffan J, Fisch RD, Prelaud P, Guaguere E, Fontaine J, Carlotti DN (2002) Randomized controlled trial of the efficacy of cyclosporine in the treatment of atopic dermatitis in dogs. *J. Am. Vet. Med. Assoc.* Aug 1 **221**(3): 370–77.

2.9   Further reading

Friedman LM, Furberg CD, DeMets DL (1998) What is the question? In: *Fundamentals of Clinical Trials*, 3rd edn, Springer-Verlag, New York, pp 16–40.
Hulley SB, Cummings SR, Browner WS, Grady DG, Newman TB (2007) Conceiving the research question. In: *Designing Clinical Research*, 3rd edn, Lippincott Williams and Wilkins, Philadelphia, pp 17–25.
Kumar R (2005) Formulating a research problem. In: *Research Methodology*, 2nd edn, Sage Publications Ltd, London, pp 39–53.
Thrusfield M (2005) Causality. In: *Veterinary Epidemiology*, 3rd edn, Blackwell Publishing, Oxford, pp 34–45.

2.10   MCQs

1 *Which of the following is the least important characteristic of a good clinical research question?*

(a) Technical feasibility.
(b) Acceptable financial and time costs.
(c) Interesting and relevant.
(d) Novel.
(e) Ethical.

2 *When selecting a secondary question which of the following factors should be considered?*

(a) Secondary questions should be specified at the design stage.
(b) Secondary questions should be chosen on a rational basis.
(c) Secondary questions should be limited in number.
(d) There should be a reasonable expectation of obtaining a significant result.
(e) All the above.

3 *What is the formal statistical description of the research question?*

(a) The null hypothesis.
(b) The alternative hypothesis.
(c) The statistical hypothesis.
(d) The research hypothesis.
(e) The formal hypothesis.

4 *What is meant by the null hypothesis in a study seeking to establish that there is a difference between two groups?*

(a) That the study hypothesis is untrue.
(b) That there is no difference between the two study groups.
(c) The results from two groups are statistically different.
(d) The research hypothesis is true.
(e) The difference between the groups is zero.

5 *Which of the following is NOT a suitable strategy when a study is not feasible because not enough subjects can be recruited?*

(a) Expand the inclusion criteria.
(b) Reduce the exclusion criteria.

(c)   Expand the sources of patients.
(d)   Lengthen the timeframe of the study.
(e)   Perform the study and then recruit a statistician to help prove statistical significance.

2.11   MCQ answers

1 (d) Although new or novel research is important, the expansion of knowledge through the repetition of clinical research is also valuable in order to increase our confidence in the original finding.

2 (e) All the factors listed are important in choosing secondary research questions.

3 (b) The experimental hypothesis is described as the alternative hypothesis. The null hypothesis is what the statistical test will attempt to prove and when rejected provides evidence that the alternative hypothesis is correct.

4 (a) The statistical test performed seeks to provide evidence that there is no difference between the two groups of statistics generated. This is the null hypothesis.

5 (e) It is always best to use a statistician during the design stage. They may help to suggest strategies to reduce the number of subjects required.

3

SAMPLING, SUBJECT SELECTION CRITERIA AND RECRUITMENT

Objectives

After reading this chapter readers should:

- be familiar with the principles of sampling in surveys, observational studies and intervention studies
- know how sampling in surveys, observational studies and intervention studies relate to internal and external validity.

3.1   Introduction

Clinical research is performed on diseased or healthy animals. It may involve studies that investigate epidemiology, diagnosis, treatment, prognosis and prevention. The methods used are surveys, observational studies and intervention studies (clinical trials). This chapter describes the sampling techniques that may be used and recruitment considerations. The treatment allocation methods that are used in clinical trials will be described in more detail in Chapter 9.

Researchers are often bound by cost, convenience and time. An appropriate representative sample of the population of interest must be identified which will provide an answer to the scientific question being investigated. The validity of generalizing from a sample to a population is crucial. The appropriate definition of the target population is paramount. If the research question involves animals with disease in medical settings then veterinary practices and veterinary hospitals are appropriate. If the scientific questions relate to treatment and prognosis the results may have generalizability; this will be less so with questions regarding diagnosis and prevalence studies. If the selection of the sample is flawed or biased then the results generated will be inaccurate and invalid.

The uncertainty of drawing inferences to other populations illustrates that generalizability is a complex and often qualitative judgement. However, by applying appropriate scientific methodology it is possible to reduce the uncertainty.

The investigator begins by specifying the clinical and population characteristics of the target population. Temporal and geographic criteria are superimposed to identify a study sample that is representative and attainable, usually within a specified budget.

3.2   Sampling

Great care and caution are required when sampling a population in veterinary medicine. The sample may not be representative of the population in general. For example, sampling animals presented at a clinic in a large urban centre may not be representative of the country as a whole. Similarly, questionnaires are widely used but bias may be introduced because responders and non-responders may not be homogeneous.

The population of subjects that meet the selection criteria will be too large and there is a need to select a sample. If we want to know the average age of a dog in the UK we could ask each dog owner and work it out. This would be expensive, time-consuming and practically impossible. We could, however, take a smaller number of representative dogs and generate an estimate of the average age of a dog in the UK. This would be quicker, cheaper and easier but the answer might be slightly different from the true age and would therefore be an estimate. Similarly, as a farm animal veterinarian I may want to know what proportion of cows are culled because of lameness in the UK. I could set up a recording system on the 19 000 dairy farms or I could select a smaller number of representative dairy farms and generate an estimate of the true figure.

The concept of sampling is an easy principle to understand but is not always easy to perform. Sampling is the process of selecting a few individuals (a sample) from a larger group (the target population) to enable an estimate or prediction to be made about a given characteristic in the target population. Sampling reduces the workload and cost of obtaining a value for the desired characteristic. The sample must be representative of the target population otherwise the outcome of the sampling will be invalid or inaccurate. The sample size, the size of the target population, the prevalence and the variation in the characteristic being measured will influence the confidence intervals for the estimate derived from the sample.

The disadvantage of sampling is that you only get an estimate or prediction, which should have a confidence interval indicating the range of value with a given degree of certainty. It is a trade-off between gains and losses in time, costs and resources. Errors can also occur in the selection of a representative sample and this will result in an inaccurate result due to the error incurred. For example, if I am trying to estimate the prevalence of hyperthyroidism in the general feline population and I take my sample from referral clinics then my estimate is likely to be grossly inaccurate. Similarly, if I am interested in the prevalence of laminitis in ponies in the UK and I question members of the pony club, my sample may not be representative of the UK pony population.

3.2.1   Definitions

The total population for which you want to answer a question is called the target population. This should be the same as the study population, which is the population from which the sample is drawn. In some studies the study population may not represent the target population and generalizations are likely to be invalid, for example if information derived from livestock shows is generalized to the national population. The study population consists of elementary units which cannot be sub-divided; in veterinary clinical studies this usually consists of individual animals. Elementary units which share a common characteristic, for example sex or breed, may be grouped together into a stratum. In order to facilitate sampling, members of the study population are sometimes identified by a number or name

and placed in a list. This list is called a sampling frame and each member is a sampling unit. In a study where the herd is the sampling population the sampling frame may be composed of ear tag numbers, with each cow being a sampling unit. The group of subjects you select to obtain an estimate for the population is called the sample. The number of subjects you select is called the sample size. The method used to select the subjects is called the sampling design or sampling strategy. The results obtained from the sample are called the sample statistics. The estimates derived from the sample statistics are called the population parameters or the population mean.

3.2.2   Principles of sampling

There are three principles behind effective sampling: the first is that there will always be a small random difference between the population parameter and the sample statistic, the second is that bigger sample sizes tend to minimize this difference, and the third is that if there is considerable variation between individuals this difference is likely to be larger. Let us investigate an example that illustrates the first principle. Suppose there are four grower pigs in pen 32. Our clinical question is 'What is the average weight of a pig in pen 32?'. The weights of the individual pigs in pen 32 are Pig A 18 kg, Pig B 20 kg, Pig C 23 kg and Pig D 25 kg. We can find out their average weight by summing their individual weights (18 + 20 + 23 + 25 = 86 kg) and dividing the total by 4 (86/4 = 21.5 kg).

Suppose we select a sample of two individuals to make an estimate of the average weight of the four pigs. There are six possible sample combinations of two pigs:

1. A (18) + B (20) = 38/2 = 19.0 kg
2. A (18) + C (23) = 41/2 = 20.5 kg
3. A (18) + D (25) = 43/2 = 21.5 kg
4. B (20) + C (23) = 43/2 = 21.5 kg
5. B (20) + D (25) = 45/2 = 22.5 kg
6. C (23) + D (25) = 48/2 = 24.0 kg

Sample number	Sample average (1)	Population average (2)	Sampling error (1−2)
1	19.0	21.5	−2.5
2	20.5	21.5	−1.5
3	21.5	21.5	0.0
4	21.5	21.5	0.0
5	22.5	21.5	+1.0
6	24.0	21.5	+2.5

In most cases there will be a difference between the sample statistics and the true population parameter even when the selection methodology is appropriate. This is due to the probabilities of selection.

Taking the same example but this time using three pig samples we will now illustrate the second principle. There are four possible combinations of three pigs:

1. A (18) + B (20) + C (23) = 61/3 = 20.33 kg
2. A (18) + B (20) + D (25) = 63/3 = 21.00 kg
3. A (18) + C (23) + D (25) = 66/3 = 22.00 kg
4. B (20) + C (23) + D (25) = 68/3 = 22.67 kg

Sample number	Sample average (1)	Population average (2)	Sampling error (1−2)
1	20.33	21.5	−1.17
2	21.00	21.5	−0.50
3	22.00	21.5	+0.5
4	22.67	21.5	+1.17

The greater the sample size the more accurate the estimate of the true population parameter will be.

To illustrate the third principle the range of weights is increased so that weights of the pigs are Pig A 18 kg, Pig B 26 kg, Pig C 32 kg and Pig D 40 kg. The range of the sampling error would then be −7.00 kg to +7.00 kg for the two-pig samples and −3.67 kg to +3.67 kg for the three-pig samples. These ranges are greater than in the first example. This introduces the third principle.

The greater the differences between individuals in the population with regard to the charac-teristic being measured the greater will be the difference between the sample statistic and the true population parameter. The greater the variation the higher will be the standard error for a given sample size. The confidence intervals will be wider, indicating our increasing uncertainty as to the accurate value of the population parameter.

The aim of the sampling procedure is to achieve the best precision for the sample size used and to avoid bias in the selection of the sample. Bias may arise from non-participation of the population, inappropriate selection of the sample and the use of non-random methods.

3.2.3   Probability sampling

Probability sampling provides a rigorous method of ensuring the validity of generalizing the findings from a sample to a population in the form of statistical significance and confidence intervals.

To be representative each subject in the population should have an equal and independent chance of selection in the sample. This is known as random sampling. Difficulties arise if a sub-population refuses or cannot participate in the study. This may make the sample unrepresenta-tive. Dependency may arise if an owner insists that all of his or her dogs participate or none.

Random samples represent the sampling population and inferences drawn from these samples can be generalized to the sampling population. Random samples are a prerequisite when applying statistics that are based on the theory of probability.

Computer programs or a table of random numbers are most commonly used to identify the sample members. Alternatively, each subject in the population can be allocated a number and the numbers drawn blindly out of a hat. It is important to remember that if this method is used the numbers should be replaced after they have been drawn and their numbers noted.

If a number is subsequently drawn twice it is replaced and the draw repeated until the sample size is obtained. This is to ensure there is the same probability of being selected for each individual in the population at each draw. If the numbers drawn are not replaced, the remaining individuals have an increased probability of being sampled.

3.2.4   Random sampling designs

Simple random sampling

Each element or subject is given an equal and independent chance of selection. The population is defined. The sample size (*n*) is defined. A method of random selection is used to identify *n* in the population.

Systematic sampling

This method is sometimes used in production animal research (Fig. 3.1). Using a list of animals or a line of animals in a chute a sample is selected by periodic counting or by selecting sampling units at equal intervals. For example, every fourth animal may be selected for the sample or alternate animals may be selected to join an experimental or control group. Bias is possible although unusual with systematic sampling and it is not a foolproof randomization technique although it is commonly used.

Stratified random sampling

Stratified sampling is used to reduce the variability and increase the accuracy of the estimate for a given sample size. The population is stratified so that the subpopulation within a stratum is more homogeneous. Stratification may use characteristics such as age, breed or the severity of a clinical condition. The sampling population is separated into groups (strata) that do not overlap. The required number of subjects is then randomly selected from each stratum. There are two types of stratified sampling: proportionate and disproportionate. Proportionate sampling is

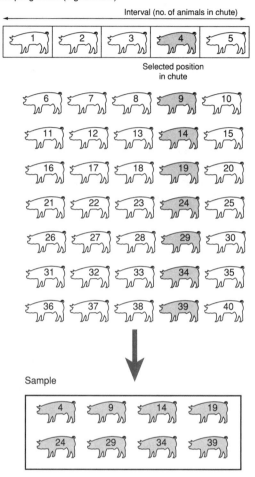

Figure 3.1 Illustration of the use of systematic sampling in a clinical study.

the most desirable method of stratified random sampling.

Proportionate sampling

Proportionate sampling randomly selects subjects from each stratum according to their relative proportions within the population. For example, consider the recruitment of a total of *n* samples: if stratum A contained 50% of the relevant population then 0.5 of the samples in *n* would be randomly selected from this stratum.

If stratum B contained 25% of the relevant population then 0.25 of the samples in *n* would be randomly selected from this stratum and so on. This could be used if we wished to estimate the regional prevalence of a disease amongst cattle: herd sampling could be proportional to the representation of beef and dairy cattle in the sampling population.

Disproportionate sampling

Disproportionate sampling randomly selects equal numbers of subjects from each stratum irrespective of the size of the strata.

Cluster sampling

Stratification becomes difficult when populations are large and geographically dispersed. In these situations cluster sampling may be used. The population is divided into groups called clusters. Simple random sampling is then performed within each cluster. In studies that have a hierarchical component multiple-stage clustering can be used. For example, if we wanted to review the treatments used for pyoderma in dogs we could randomly select veterinary practices as our clusters and examine the records within each of these practices.

Multiple-stage clustering can be used in populations that are composed of subgroups, such as pig pens in a finishing unit. A random sample of pig farms is first selected from the population of interest. A random sample of pens within each pig farm is then selected. Next a random sample of individuals from each pig pen is selected.

3.2.5 Non-random/non-probability sampling

These designs are used when the number of subjects in a population is either unknown or cannot be individually identified. The selection of subjects is dependent on other factors. There are four designs that may be used, depending on the circumstances.

Quota sampling

Ease of access to the sample population is the paramount consideration with this design. It is also driven by the ability to recognize a given characteristic in the target population such as breed, overweight dogs or chronically lame cows. Whenever a qualifying subject is identified it is recruited into the study until a target sample size is reached. Because the sample is not randomly selected the findings cannot be generalized to the population. This can be a useful technique for hypothesis generation.

Accidental sampling

This method is used when the ease and convenience of sampling are the overriding factors. No attempt is made to identify qualifying characteristics. A pet food company may be interested in which cat food people feed to their cats. The people asked may or may not have a cat.

Judgemental or purposive sampling

The object of the study may be to define an accurate clinical profile of a new and emerging disease (e.g. BSE in 1985). The people considered to have the required information can be targeted (cattle veterinarians). This approach is useful in descriptive studies of diseases about which little is known. Judgemental approaches have also been used to identify representative samples from a target population. It is acknowledged that this approach is flawed.

Snowball sampling

People are targeted who may have the information required by the study. They are then asked to identify other people in the organization who then become part of the sample. This method is useful to gain insights into communication patterns, contact networks, decision-making and diffusion of knowledge within a group.

These survey-sampling designs are shown in Fig. 3.2.

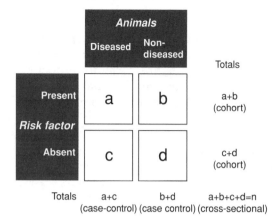

Figure 3.2 Information that is pre-determined before the start of cohort, case-control and cross-sectional studies.

3.3 Surveys

Surveys are used to measure the prevalence or magnitude of a parameter (e.g. weight or milk yield) in a target population. A representative sample of the target population is surveyed.

3.4 Observational clinical studies and clinical trials

There are three main types of observational study: cohort, case-control and cross-sectional studies (Fig. 3.3).

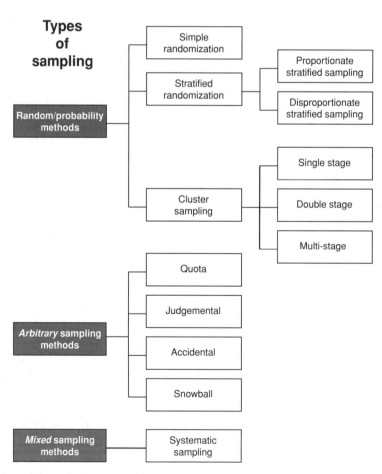

Figure 3.3 Sampling techniques used in surveys.

In cohort studies (A + B) and (C + D) are pre-determined before the start of the study. In case-control studies (A + C) and (B + D) are pre-determined before the start of the study. In cross-sectional studies only *n* is pre-determined before the start of the study.

3.4.1 Observational clinical studies

Cohort studies

In cohort studies a group (cohort) of animals exposed to a specified factor and a group not exposed to the specified factor are selected and observed over time for the development of a defined disease. An example of this type of study is healthy neonatal calves with adequate and inadequate passive transfer of colostral immuno-globulins and their subsequent development of diarrhoea. The animals selected for the groups have an inclusion criteria based on the presence or absence of a specified risk factor and the absence of disease. The target population is the population represented by the groups.

Case-control studies

In a case-control study a group of diseased animals and a group of non-diseased animals are selected and the presence or absence of a specified risk factor(s) recorded. Cats with and without lymphosarcoma may be tested for the presence or absence of feline leukaemia virus (FeLV). The animals selected for the groups have inclusion criteria based on the presence or absence of disease. The target population is the population represented by the groups.

Cross-sectional studies

In cross-sectional studies the presence or absence of a specified disease and factor in each individual of a sample taken from the target population is determined. A sample of bitches from a target population could be classified according to whether they have been spayed or not

and whether they have developed physiological urinary incontinence or not. The prevalence of disease can be determined from the data collected. At the beginning of the study only the sample size is known.

3.4.2 Clinical trials

Veterinary clinical trials are systematic studies that investigate the effects of a treatment on animal subjects. A sample of the target population is required (Fig. 3.4). The experimental unit is the smallest independent unit to which a treatment is allocated. This may be an udder quarter on a cow, an individual animal or a group of pigs in a pen. The experimental population is the population in which the trial is conducted. There is usually at least one treatment group and one control group. The experimental design needs to be appropriate to ensure internal validity, i.e. the observed differences between the experimental and control groups are due to the treatment effects. The experimental population should be representative of the target population to ensure the results are externally valid, i.e. there is generalizability of the results to the target population. The selection of the subjects for the control and treatment groups should be based on inclusion and external criteria. Informed consent must be obtained and the experiment should be legal and ethical.

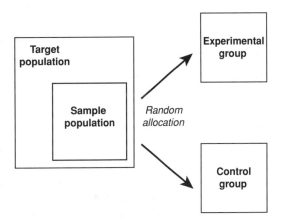

Figure 3.4 Sampling for a clinical trial.

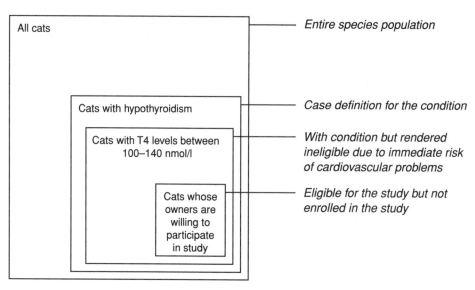

Figure 3.5 Selection of a study sample from a target population.

Selection criteria

Inclusion criteria are the requirements that a subject must fulfil to be allowed to enter a study. These are usually devised to ensure that the subject has the appropriate disease and that the animal or owner is the type of subject that the researchers wish to study. Inclusion criteria should not simply be the opposites of the exclusion criteria.

Exclusion criteria are the reasons why a subject should not be enrolled into the study. These are usually reasons of safety and should not simply be the opposites of the inclusion criteria. Recruitment is the process of enrolling subjects in a study.

It is important that inclusion and exclusion criteria are used consistently throughout the recruitment of subjects, and that the criteria are sufficiently detailed to enable consistency of interpretation.

The inclusion criteria should define populations that are relevant to the research question. They may include signalment, such as species, age, breed, lactating or adult, clinical characteristics, such as the presence of the target disease (and possible stage of disease, e.g. mild, moderate, severe, acute, chronic), geographical location (country) and temporal framework (study period 12 months). The task of specifying clinical characteristics often involves difficult judgements about what factors are important to the clinical research question and how to define them.

The exclusion criteria may specify subsets of the population because there is a high likelihood of being lost to follow-up (potential cull dairy cows), being at high risk from side effects (pregnant) or characteristics that make it unethical to withhold the additional treatments. Exclusion criteria may improve the feasibility of a study at the cost of generalizability so researchers should use them sparingly. Before starting the study the reviewer should consider whether the exclusion criteria will invalidate the generalizability of the study. The process is illustrated in Fig. 3.5.

Recruitment

Recruitment can be a difficult process. There is a need to consider accessibility, whether or not the sample represents the target population, whether or not sufficient numbers can be recruited for the study to have sufficient power to answer the scientific question and whether or not the dropout rate will be too high once the study period begins.

Owners that are difficult to contact and those who refuse to participate once they are included in the trial tend to be different from owners who do respond, which compromises the generalizability of the study. Recruiting sufficient numbers of subjects is one of the most difficult tasks in veterinary clinical research.

Sampling and applicability

The term 'applicability' refers to the extent to which the results of a study are relevant to, or can be applied in, clinical settings other than the study and is sometimes known as generalizability. Applicability is made up of two components: how biologically similar patients are and whether the process of the intervention can be replicated. The method of sampling will influence how biologically applicable the study is and the details of the intervention and the setting will determine the process application. The details and resources needed should be clearly stated and the intervention must be explicit in order to ensure that the study could be replicated.

Sampling is the method that is used to select and recruit the subjects of the study. The selection criteria are based on inclusion and exclusion criteria. These criteria define the sample(s). If very strict criteria are used to provide a homogeneous sample the differences are more likely to be due to a risk factor or treatment. However, the results of a study with strict entry and exclusion criteria will apply to fewer animals than if less strict criteria were used.

There are financial and time pressures to reduce the number of subjects but at the same time it is desirable that the results are applicable to as many patients as possible in as many clinical settings as possible, which tends to be achieved by using a relatively large sample.

3.5   The calculation of sample size

This is described in Chapter 6.

3.6   Summary

1. Sampling is an important concept in clinical research.
2. Appropriate sampling allows a researcher to make inferences about a larger population using a smaller sample with a relatively small cost in time and effort. However, the sampling itself may introduce a source of error. When a sample is not sufficiently representative for the research question being investigated, the results may not provide a genuine reflection of the sampled population.
3. The first step in the study design is to define the target population using a set of inclusion criteria that determine the population and the clinical characteristics of subjects appropriate to the research question, and a carefully considered set of exclusion criteria that define animals that it would be inappropriate or unethical to include in the study.
4. The next stage is to design an approach to sampling the population. The use of all clinical cases is often a good choice in clinical research, with strict adherence to exclusions (i.e. not excluding cases if they are inconvenient). Simple random sampling can be used to reduce the size of the sample if necessary, and other probability samples (stratified and cluster) may be appropriate.
5. The total number of cases or subjects must be sufficient to meet the statistical needs of the study in order for a conclusion to be drawn from the study results.

3.7   Further reading

Friedman LM, Furberg CD, DeMets DL (1998) Study population. In: *Fundamentals of Clinical Trials*, 3rd edn, Springer-Verlag, New York, pp 30–39.

Hulley SB, Cummings SR, Browner WS, Grady DG, Newman TB (2007) Choosing the study subjects: specification, sampling and recruitment. In: *Designing Clinical Research*, 3rd edn, Lippincott Williams and Wilkins, Philadelphia, pp 27–36.

Kumar R (2005) Sampling. In: *Research Methodology*, 2nd edn, Sage Publications Ltd, London, pp 161–84.

McGovern DPB, Valori RM, Summerskill WSM, Levi M (2001) *Sampling and Applicability in Key Topics in Evidence-based Medicine*, BIOS Scientific Publications Ltd, Oxford, pp 130–32.

Smith RD (2006) Statistical significance: sampling strategies. In: *Veterinary Clinical Epidemiology*, 3rd edn, CRC Press, London, pp 151–6.

Thrusfield M (2005) Surveys. In: *Veterinary Epidemiology*, 3rd edn, Blackwell Publishing, Oxford, pp 228–42.

Thrusfield M (2005) Observational studies. In: *Veterinary Epidemiology*, 3rd edn, Blackwell Publishing, Oxford, pp 266–84.

Thrusfield (2005) Clinical trials. In: *Veterinary Epidemiology*, 3rd edn, Blackwell Publishing, Oxford, pp 289–302.

3.8 MCQs

1 **Sampling is used because:**

(a) it gives the same answer as measuring the target population
(b) it gives reliable results
(c) it requires no planning
(d) it is quick and easy to do
(e) it provides an estimate whilst reducing the time and cost.

2 **The target population:**

(a) should be the same as the study population
(b) is different from the study population
(c) is a sample of the study population
(d) is the sample to be taken
(e) is the population not sampled.

3 **Differences between the sample statistic and the target population parameter value are due to:**

(a) sample size
(b) probabilities of selection

(c) inappropriate selection of samples
(d) individual variation in the parameter
(e) all of the above.

4 **Simple random sampling means:**

(a) each subject in the target population has an equal chance of selection
(b) each subject in the target population has an independent chance of selection
(c) each subject in the target population has an equal and independent chance of selection
(d) each subject in the target population may be selected
(e) each subject in the study population is selected.

5 **Proportionate sampling means:**

(a) randomly selecting equal numbers from each stratum
(b) randomly selecting unequal numbers from each stratum
(c) randomly selecting subjects from each stratum according to its relative proportion within the population
(d) selecting a proportion of the study population
(e) selecting every nth subject from the population.

6 **Clusters are:**

(a) the same as strata
(b) subjects that share a characteristic
(c) a group of subjects that are randomly dispersed in the population
(d) a randomly selected subpopulation that can be clearly defined and is usually located in one place
(e) subjects that are interdependent.

7 **Snowballing is:**

(a) a randomized method of selecting samples
(b) a method that may be useful in defining contact network structures
(c) a selection method that is self selecting
(d) a useful method to identify a target population
(e) a method of reducing errors in sampling.

8 *Using the table below indicate what is determined before the start of a cohort study.*

	Diseased animals	Non-diseased animals	Total
Risk factor present	A	B	A + B
Risk factor absent	C	D	C + D
Total	A + C	B + D	A + B + C + D = n

(a) (A + B) and (C + D)
(b) (A + C) and (B + D)
(c) n
(d) A + B
(e) C + D.

9 *Inclusion criteria are:*

(a) the requirements that a subject must fulfil to enter a study
(b) the parameter that is being measured
(c) the inverse of the exclusion criteria
(d) the same as the recruitment process
(e) subjects who want to join the study.

10 *Applicability (generalizability) is:*

(a) the extent the results of a study are relevant to a given population
(b) the usefulness of the results in general terms
(c) the results expected if the outcomes were applied to the general population
(d) the cost benefit of the study
(e) the application of the results to all species.

3.9 MCQ answers

1 (e); 2 (a); 3 (e); 4 (c); 5 (c); 6 (d); 7 (b); 8 (a); 9 (a); 10 (a)

VARIABLES

Objectives

Objectives

After reading this chapter readers should:

- understand the type of measurements of a variable that are required to describe the phenomena being studied
- understand how to optimize the precision and accuracy of these measurements.

4.1 Introduction

'Variable' is the mathematical term for a characteristic or property of something that is being measured, for example dullness may be a variable to which a value is attached to describe pain in an animal and blood urea nitrogen may be a variable that is measured to describe renal function. Data are produced by measuring and attaching a value to, the variable. The choice of a measurement scale influences the information content of the measurement. Minimizing the measurement error will improve the validity of the estimate derived from the sample. The aim is to select variables that can describe the phenomenon of interest and design measurements that are precise (free from random error) and accurate (free from systematic error).

The choice of a variable affects the way in which the data produced can be analysed, what statistical tests can be applied, what interpretations can be made, how the data can be presented and what conclusions can be drawn. The selection of the most appropriate variable is vital in the experimental design. It determines whether the study is predominantly qualitative or quantitative.

4.2 Types of variable

It is important when designing a study to identify appropriate variables. Sometimes it is useful to consider the different types of variables that may need to be measured.

When investigating causal or association relationships three sets of variables may operate (Fig. 4.1): independent variables (assumed cause), dependent variables (assumed effect) and extraneous variables (influencing factors).

To explain these variables, suppose you want to study the relationship between ingestion of abnormal prions (independent variable) and the development of scrapie in sheep (dependent variable). Factors such as the genotype, age of sheep and dose rate ingested (extraneous variable) will influence the development of clinical scrapie. Careful consideration of the different types of variable and how they will be measured is an important step in the conceptual stage of the study design.

In controlled experiments the independent (cause) variable may be introduced or manipulated by the researcher. These are called active variables. Attribute variables are variables that cannot be controlled, changed or manipulated. In a study to investigate the response of pyoderma in dogs to a given antibiotic the antibiotic would be the active variable. The weight, diet

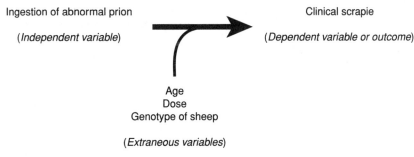

Figure 4.1 Types of variable.

Table 4.1   Characteristics and examples of measurement scales.

Type	Measurement scale	Example	Characteristics
Qualitative (Categorical)	Nominal	Breed	Unordered categories
	Nominal	Male/female Alive/dead	Dichotomous/binary
	Ordinal	Mild, moderate, severe pain	Ordered categories with intervals that are not quantifiable
Quantitative	Discrete (counts)	Number of puppies in litter	Can only have one of an ordered specified set of values
	Continuous (interval)	Temperature	Ordered ranked spectrum of quantifiable intervals
	Continuous (ratio)	Weight	Ordered ranked spectrum of quantifiable intervals but has a fixed starting point, e.g. zero

and exercise regime may be attribute variables that cannot be easily manipulated. The term predictor variable is used to indicate a variable that can be used to predict the value of an outcome variable.

4.3   Measurement scales

Some types of variable provide more information and informative statistics than others therefore adding power to the study and reducing the sample size requirement.

Table 4.1 provides a classification of the measurement scales that can be used to measure variables.

4.3.1   *Qualitative variables*

Categorical variables

Categorical variables generate data that describe the number in each category. Categorical variables have two or more categories and can be further subdivided into nominal variables (unranked) or ordinal variables (ranked).

Nominal variables

The nominal scale is used to classify objects or subjects. Members of the same class must have the same nominated characteristic. Nominal variables tend to be qualitative with no numer-

ical relationship to one another, e.g. breed and coat colour. There are no ordered or numerical relationships between Labrador, blood hound and cocker spaniel. These are unrelated subgroups.

Some nominal variables can only be grouped into two categories and are known as dichotomous or binary variables. Examples include dead/alive, improved/not improved, male/female.

Ordinal variables

Ordinal (ordered, ranked) variables have multiple categories that have an order, for example mild, moderate or severe. They consist of classes or subgroups that have some sort of ranking system or inherent order to them, for example lameness and heart murmurs. There is a clearly ordered or ranked relationship but there is not a well-defined mathematical relationship between different values, for example condition scoring cow A with score 4 does not mean cow A is twice as fat as cow B with a score of 2 but it is fatter than cow B.

4.3.2   *Quantitative variables*

Discrete variables

Discrete continuous variables, such as the number of dogs in a household, exist as integer counts.

Continuous variables

Intervals

Continuous variables have quantified intervals within a range which may be an infinite scale of values. This type of variable is rich in information. Examples of continuous variables are weight, age, body temperature and blood glucose.

Ratio scale

The zero point of a ratio scale is fixed. It is an absolute scale. The measurement of age, height, weight and the milk yield of two individuals can all be expressed on a ratio scale.

4.3.3   Hierarchy of variable types

Variable types can be viewed as a hierarchy in that a variable can always be analysed as if it were a type further down the hierarchy, but not vice versa:

continuous > ordinal > categorical > binary

For example, we can transpose a continuous variable such as blood urea nitrogen into an ordinal scale of high, intermediate, low and then into a binary scale of normal/abnormal using appropriate cut-off points. There is loss of information by doing so but the result may improve clinical interpretation or allow a non-parametric statistical analysis to be performed, which would not be justified using a continuous scale.

4.3.4   Choosing a measurement scale

The continuous variable contains more information and the result is a study with more power than other scales of measure. Even if the study outcome is dichotomous, for example the mortality rate in low birth weight piglets, it is still best to collect the data as a continuous variable so that the data can be explored by changing the cut-off points of the birth weights. Similarly,

with an ordinal scale sometimes it is better to use several categories even if the outcomes are collapsed into fewer categories for the final analysis. Many clinical abnormalities are difficult to describe with categories or numbers. Clear definitions and consistency of categorization are important. Measurements need to generate useful data within time and cost budgets.

4.3.5   Refinement

This is the degree of detail used in a measurement; increasing the number of decimal places used in a measurement makes it a more refined measurement. Hypocalcaemia is a more refined diagnosis than a cow with flaccid paralysis. Precision can mean the same as refinement: the meaning of precision when used in the context of the measurement is used to indicate the consistency of a series of repeated measurements.

4.3.6   Other scales of measurement

Analogue scales

Analogue scales use a straight line with both ends having a description of the two extreme values of the variable. Lameness, pain and alertness can be assessed in this way. This is really a method of measuring a variable using a subjective ordinal scale.

Composite measure scales

These have been used to assess pain in farm animals. They numerically combine a range of nominal, ordinal, interval and ratio variable measures. It is important there is content and construct validity. Content validity is how well the scale represents the range of features associated with the phenomenon of interest and construct validity is how adequately the scale represents the qualities of the phenomenon of interest.

4.4   Precision and accuracy

Precision and accuracy are important aspects of measurements. Poor precision will reduce the power of an experiment to demonstrate a difference and poor accuracy will result in invalid conclusions.

4.4.1   Precision (reproducibility, reliability, consistency)

Definitions

Reliable: produces similar results when the technique is repeated.
Repeatability: agreement between sets of observations made on the same animals by the same observer.
Reproducibility: agreement between sets of observations on the same animals by different observers.

A very precise measurement is one that is reproducible with nearly the same value each time the measurement is repeated. The more precise the measurement the greater the statistical power at a given sample size. Precision is affected by random error (chance). The greater the error the less precise the measurement becomes. There are three main sources of error: observer variability, subject variability and instrument variability.

Observer variability refers to the variability of measurement due to the observer. This may involve errors in observation or the use of instrumentation. Instrument variability refers to variability in the measurement caused by faults in the instrument. Reagents, temperature, worn parts and electrical faults may all produce variability. Subject variability refers to intrinsic biological variation in the subjects caused by some factor such as activity or feed.

Assessing precision

Precision is assessed as the consistency of repeated measurements. This can be performed as follows:

- within-observer reproducibility: a single observer performs repeated measurements on a set of subjects

- between-observer reproducibility: different observers perform repeated measurements on a set of subjects
- within-instrument reproducibility: a single instrument is used for repeated measurements on a set of subjects
- between-instrument reproducibility: different instruments are used for repeated measurements on a set of subjects.

The reproducibility of continuous variables can be expressed with the statistic within-subject standard deviation. For categorical variables percentage agreement and the kappa statistic are often used.

Strategies to improve precision

Standardizing measurement methods

Specific written protocols can help to standardize the methods used to measure the variable and hence reduce observer variability.

Training and assessing the observers

Training will improve the consistency of measurement techniques and reduce inter-observer variability.

Refining the instruments

Mechanical and electronic equipment can be serviced and set to reduce instrument variability.

Automating the measurements

Minimizing the observer inputs to the process of measurement will reduce errors caused by the observer using the instrumentation incorrectly.

Repetition

The effect of random error from any source is reduced by repeating the measurement and using the mean of the values.

Table 4.2 Examples of strategies that can be used to reduce random error and increase precision.

	Example	Source of error	Reduction of error
Standardization of measurement protocols	Body condition scores for cattle	Observer (subjective assessment)	Use ultrasound machines to measure lumbar fat thickness
Training of observer	Assessment of post-operative pain in dogs	Inexperience	Use a training video
Refining the instrument	Study on conception rates in cattle	Manual detection of pregnancy under 40 days	Use an ultrasound machine
Automating the instrument	Heart rate measurements in cats with hyperthyroidism	Measuring the ECG print out	Use computer-generated counts
Repeating the measurement	Mean weight change of a group of animals on a given diet	Sample may not be representative	Repeat the sample

Table 4.2 indicates some of the strategies that can be used to reduce random error.

If low precision is a perceived problem then assessment of which strategies to adopt should be performed. Factors that will influence the choice will include the importance of the variable, the size of the problem, the perceived source of the error and the feasibility and cost of implementing change. In general, providing written protocols and training should be a standard procedure. Repetition of the measurement will always increase the precision.

4.4.2 Accuracy (validity)

The accuracy of a variable is the degree to which it actually represents what it is intended to represent. An inaccurate variable will give rise to low internal and external validity. Table 4.3 and Fig. 4.2 illustrate the difference between accuracy and precision.

Accuracy is an inverse function of systematic error. Systematic error is the same as bias and bias can occur due to the observer, the subject or the instruments used in the measurements. Observer bias occurs when there is an error when using the measuring instruments or in the interpretation of an observation or in the manner in which an interview was conducted. Subject bias may occur when owners give biased information regarding their animals, such as the amount of exercise an animal receives or the amount of food it eats. Instrument bias, such as incorrect calibration, may produce consistently lower or higher

Table 4.3 Comparison of accuracy and precision.

	Precision	Accuracy
Interpretation	High precision: variable has the same value with repeated measures Low precision: the variable has widely dispersed values with repeated measures	High accuracy: measurement is close to the variable value Low accuracy: the measurement value is not close to the variable value
Measurement	Compare repeated measurements	Compare to a gold standard
Reduced by	Random error	Systematic error (bias)

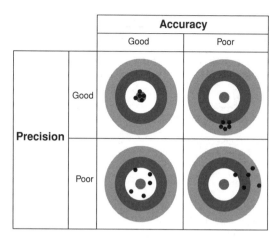

Figure 4.2 Accuracy and precision expressed as a shooting target.

results. Accuracy can be assessed by comparing the result to a gold standard.

Assessment of accuracy

Accuracy is expressed in different ways depending on whether the measurement is on a continuous or categorical scale. For example, the accuracy of an equine weight band used to estimate the weight of a horse by measuring the girth circumference on a continuous scale may be expressed as a correlation line. The accuracy of a test to classify animals into diseased or not diseased categories can be expressed as the specificity and sensitivity on a categorical scale when compared to a gold standard.

Strategies to increase accuracy

Accuracy may be increased by implementing the following: using protocols to standardize the measuring methods, training the observers, automating, refining and calibrating the instruments used in measuring, blinding the observer and making the subjects unaware that they are being observed. The importance of the variable, the potential impact and the feasibility and cost of implementing the change should be consid-

ered. Table 4.4 provides examples of strategies that can be used to reduce systematic error and increase accuracy.

4.4.3   Behavioural studies

Behavioural observations require special attention when trying to assess the validity that an observation represents a phenomenon. For example, assessing post-operative pain in bitches which have been spayed may use indicators of dullness and posture. The validity of lameness as an indicator of pain in cattle with solar ulceration may be more obvious. Validity may be obtained by the measure making intuitive sense such as the lameness example; confidence in the validity will also increase if a range of indicators of the phenomenon is recorded which are likely to be related to the phenomenon. Previous published work may also provide useful measures which have been shown to have validity. For more information on measuring behaviour, *Measuring Behaviour* by Martin and Bateson is worth consulting.

4.4.4   Sensitivity and specificity of measurements

Measurements must be sensitive enough to detect differences that are important in a clinical setting. For example, measuring the number of steps taken by a lame cow when forced to walk for 5 minutes may give the same number as a non-lame cow but the distance travelled may be less. The measure used must reflect the question being asked and be sufficiently sensitive. The range of values that can be measured must be sufficient to cover the anticipated values. Ideally the measure should be specific to the variable of interest. If other factors can influence the value of the measure then differences in the variable may be difficult to detect between a treatment group and a control group. Objective measures are the most reliable with the least error and should be used if possible.

Table 4.4   Examples of strategies that can be used to reduce systematic error and increase accuracy.

	Example	Source of systematic error	Reduction of error
Standardization of measurement protocols	Body condition scores for cattle	Consistently high scores	Use photographs of the different scores
Training of observer	Assessment of post-operative pain in dogs	Consistently low scores	Use a training video
Refining the instrument	Study on conception rates in cattle	Manual detection of pregnancy under 40 days gives consistently low rates	Use an ultrasound machine
Automating the instrument	Heart rate measurements in cats with hyperthyroidism	Inaccurate measurements of heart rate from ECG print out	Use computer-generated counts
Repeating the measurement	Mean weight change of a group of animals on a given diet	Sample not representative Sample is composed of the first easiest six pigs to be caught	Give the pigs numbers and randomly select the sample
Blinding	Treatment of canine arthritis with a test analgesic drug Comparison is with control group that receives no drug	Owner appraisal over-estimates the effect of the drug	Give placebo to control group
Calibration of the instrument	Rumen fluid pH measurement	Instrument not recalibrated between recordings	Calibrate the meter between recordings with standardized solutions

4.4.5   *Measurements on stored materials and records*

Records can be used to measure clinical signs, temporal changes, treatment responses, weight, longevity and breed prevalence. Stored material may include biopsies, blood samples, bone, urine and radiographs.

4.5   Summary

1. Variables may be described as:
   - continuous: quantified on an infinite scale
   - discrete: quantified on a finite scale
   - categorical: classified in categories.
   Categorical variables are further classified as nominal (unordered) or ordinal (ordered). Variables that have only two categories are called dichotomous.

2. Variables that contain more information permit smaller sample sizes. In order of preference the type of variable that should be used if possible is: continuous, discrete, ordered categorical, nominal and dichotomous.

3. The precision of a measurement (i.e. the reproducibility of replicated measures) is another major influence on power and sample size. Precision is reduced by random error (i.e. chance) from three sources of variability: the observer, the method of measurement and the subject.

4. There are two strategies that help to increase precision:
   - define and standardize methods in an operations manual
   - train and certify staff involved in collecting data.

Other strategies that may be employed are improving the data collection instruments, using automation when possible and using the mean of repeated measurements.

5. The accuracy of a measurement (i.e. the degree to which it actually measures the characteristic it is supposed to measure) is a major determinant of inferring correct conclusions. Accuracy is reduced by systematic error (i.e. bias) from three sources: the observer, the method of measurement and the subject.

6. The strategies for increasing accuracy include all those listed for precision with the exception of repetition. In addition, accuracy is enhanced by calibration, and (in comparisons between groups) by blinding.

7. Each measurement should be sensitive, specific, appropriate and objective, and they should produce a range of values.

4.6   Further reading

Hulley SB, Cummings SR, Browner WS, Grady DG, Newman TB (2007) Planning the measurements: precision and accuracy. In: *Designing Clinical Research*, 3rd edn, Lippincott Williams and Wilkins, Philadelphia, pp 37–49.

Kumar R (2005) Sampling. In: *Research Methodology*, 2nd edn, Sage Publications Ltd, London, pp 161–206.

Martin P, Bateson P (1993) *Measuring Behaviour*, 2nd edn, Cambridge University Press, Cambridge.

Smith RD (2006) Defining the limits of normality. In: *Veterinary Clinical Epidemiology*, 3rd edn, CRC Press, London, pp 13–32.

Thrusfield M (2005) The nature of data. In: *Veterinary Epidemiology*, 3rd edn, Blackwell Publishing, Oxford, pp 152–67.

4.7   MCQs

1 *Continuous variables are:*

(a) quantified on an infinite scale
(b) classified in unordered categories
(c) classified into ordered categories
(d) termed dichotomous
(e) quantified on a finite scale.

2 *Discrete variables are:*

(a) quantified on an infinite scale
(b) classified in unordered categories
(c) classified into ordered categories
(d) termed dichotomous
(e) quantified on a finite scale.

3 *Nominal categorical variables are:*

(a) quantified on an infinite scale
(b) classified in unordered categories
(c) classified into ordered categories
(d) termed dichotomous
(e) quantified on a finite scale.

4 *Ordinal categorical variables are:*

(a) quantified on an infinite scale
(b) classified in unordered categories
(c) classified into ordered categories
(d) termed dichotomous
(e) quantified on a finite scale.

5 *Which type of variable contains more information and will allow a reduction in sample size?*

(a) Nominal variables.
(b) Dichotomous variables.
(c) Ordered categorical variables.
(d) Discrete variables.
(e) Continuous variables.

6 *Precision is:*

(a) reduced by systematic error
(b) increased by random error
(c) the reproducibility of replicate measures
(d) increased by systematic error
(e) the same as accuracy.

7 *Accuracy is:*

(a) reduced by systematic error
(b) increased by random error
(c) the reproducibility of replicate measures
(d) reduced by systematic error
(e) the same as precision.

8 *A strategy that will increase precision but not accuracy is:*

(a) repetition
(b) training observers
(c) use of standardized protocols
(d) refining instruments
(e) automating instruments.

9 *Accuracy of a measurement can best be assessed by:*

(a) comparing it to a gold standard
(b) repeated measures
(c) measuring the precision

(d) repeating the experiment
(e) using instruments.

10 *Precision can be best assessed by:*

(a) comparing it to a gold standard
(b) repeated measures
(c) measuring the accuracy
(d) measuring the sensitivity and specificity
(e) using instruments.

4.8 MCQ answers

1 (a); 2 (e); 3 (b); 4 (c); 5 (e); 6 (c); 7 (d); 8 (a); 9 (a); 10 (b)

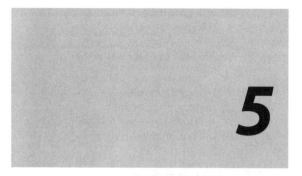

5

INTRODUCING STATISTICS

Objectives

After reading this chapter readers should understand the following underlying statistical principles:

- type I and type II errors
- magnitude of effect
- alpha and beta probabilities, and power
- *P* value.

5.1 Introduction

This chapter introduces some statistical principles that need to be considered during the design phase of clinical research projects. The main objective that needs to be achieved is an estimate of the number of animals or samples that, should the hypothesis turn out to be correct, will yield the 'holy grail' of research, a statistically significant result.

The hypothesis that is being tested will dictate which statistical test should be used, although investigators will have to understand the nature of the parameters being measured (e.g. the type of variable and their independence – something that is not always obvious). In order to calculate the sample size we need to know which statistical test is being used, by how much the parameters would normally vary (e.g. relatively little in the case of plasma sodium levels or quite a lot in the case of somatic cell counts in dairy cows) and finally the effect size that we want to be able to detect. These steps in the study design are summarized in Fig. 5.1.

Before progressing too far down this path we need to understand a few basic statistical principles. Few of us derive much pleasure from the study of statistics as a leisure time activity, and clinical researchers will often include a statistician in the research team. However, just as even the least mechanically minded motorist will benefit from some basic understanding of how a motor car works (i.e. the need for petrol, oil and water, and what happens when they run out), it is extremely valuable for clinical researchers

to acquire some basic statistical knowledge and understanding.

5.2 Statistical principles

If we took a number of individuals from a herd of cows and randomly assigned each of them to one of two equally sized groups and then measured their milk yields at the next milking we would not expect them to be identical, although we would be surprised if there was a large difference between the two groups. We would expect the results to be similar but common sense tells us that there is a high possibility that a few extra high- or low-yielding cows would end up in one or other of the groups. We expect to find a difference, but it should be a small 'insignificant' difference.

If we separated the cows on the basis of age and put all the heifers in one group and the remainder of the cows in the other group, we would expect the average yield in the heifers to be lower due to their relative immaturity. Our hypothesis would be that heifers produce less milk.

Our study would be designed to test our hypothesis. A commonly used and appropriate analogy is the judicial system's attempt to test a defendant's innocence in a courtroom trial. The jury starts with the assumption of innocence, i.e. the defendant did not perform the crime. After considering the evidence the jury must decide if they should reject this presumption. Rejection of the presumption is not based on the existence of any evidence but on the weight of evidence breaching a notional threshold of 'beyond reasonable doubt'.

Returning to our study, the 'presumption of innocence' is called the null hypothesis; in this example it is that 'heifers yield the same amount of milk as older cows'. Instead of a jury trial we use a statistical test of this null hypothesis to provide evidence of 'guilt', which is described by statisticians as the alternative hypothesis. The threshold of evidence to reject the null hypothesis is the level of statistical

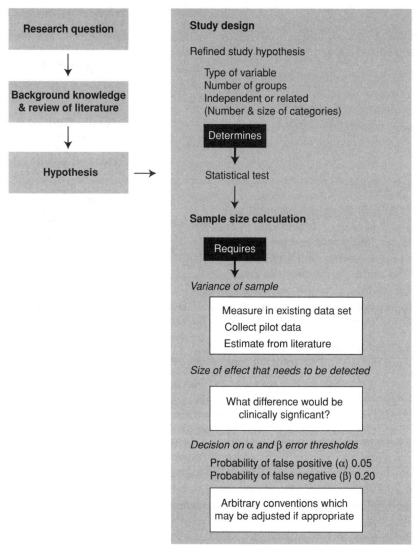

Figure 5.1 Schematic representation of the statistical decision-making process in the design of clinical studies.

significance (the *P* value, *P* < 0.05 in many of the studies described in detail later in this chapter).

5.2.1   Type I and II errors

Both juries and researchers are imperfect and both can make mistakes. In an ideal world juries would always convict the guilty and acquit the innocent. The two types of error that can be made are that a jury may convict the innocent (a false positive result) or acquit the guilty (a false negative result). In statistical terms these are referred to as type I and type II errors. A type I error is a false positive result that occurs when we incorrectly reject the null hypothesis; a type II error is a false negative result that occurs when we fail to reject the null hypothesis when we should have. These errors can never be eliminated in clinical research because of the random distribution of variables within our subjects. Each experiment has a 'lottery' component and the random distribution of subjects may lead to a lottery false positive or a lottery false negative.

It is important to distinguish type I and II errors that occur through random chance from those that are introduced through bias. If all our heifers were Friesian Holsteins (typically very high yielding dairy cows) and all our older cows were Jersey cows (typically low yielding animals), we might not get the result we expect because of the bias introduced by the confounding factor of the breeds of the cows. We minimize the effect of bias through good experimental design; we deal with false results arising from chance (type I and II errors) through the appropriate use of statistics.

There are two things that need consideration when calculating the sample size to take account of type I and II errors: the effect size and its variability.

5.2.2 Effect size

When looking at the association between a gene defect and manifestation of disease the effect may be absolute. For example, possession of two copies of the recessive gene that causes severe combined immune deficiency in Arab foals leads to the disease. Possession of a single copy produces a carrier state but the foal is otherwise normal. As you might expect, the number of animals required to demonstrate a statistically significant association is quite small. Sadly, clinical research rarely provides us with an all or nothing effect; we find ourselves looking at variables which may differ considerably between the affected or nonaffected groups or they may vary by only a small amount. Common sense suggests that when the difference is small we will require more subjects compared to situations when the difference is large.

Here is the 'Catch 22' situation (the dilemma for which there is no escape because of mutually conflicting or dependent conditions): the whole point of conducting this research is that we often don't know what the effect size is or is likely to be. However, we can come up with an estimate of what effect size we would like to detect. This might be described as the proportion of animals that had a defined clinical improvement (a reduction in the number of mastitic cows with clinical signs of mastitis) in a clinical trial of a new mastitis therapy or an average difference in a variable that is a marker of the disease state (e.g. decreased somatic cell count in the milk).

A minimum effect size is chosen or estimated to be the effect that we would like to be able to detect in the sample or one which would be the smallest clinically important effect that would be of interest.

What information can we find to help us arrive at an appropriate effect size? Firstly we can look at data from previous studies in related areas; we may be able to extrapolate from studies on different populations, species, breeds, etc. We may find data from descriptive studies (case series, surveys, etc.) that can help inform our decision. We can use data from practice or hospital records, and consult colleagues for their opinions. When no data are available the best approach may be to perform a small pilot study for the express purpose of providing data for the sample size estimation.

5.2.3 Variability

Type I and II errors are caused by the randomness of the natural world. The degree of randomness increases the likelihood of errors occurring. Some parameters we might want to measure are highly variable, such as the number of somatic cells in the milk of dairy cows, which may vary from 10 000 cells per millilitre to 1 000 000 cells per millilitre in cows not showing signs of mastitis. Other parameters, such as haemoglobin levels in healthy animals, are far less variable. Where there is a large degree of variability it is increasingly likely that the higher values from the group showing no increase in the parameter will overlap with the lower values from the group with an increase in the parameter. In studies looking at somatic cell counts we may well need much larger numbers of cows to detect a clinically important difference compared to a study attempting to detect a difference in anaemia parameters. In order to calculate the power we will need some indication of the variability and distribution of the parameters of interest in the population being studied.

How can we estimate the variability of a data set we haven't collected? If we are measuring a change in blood pressure, leucocytes or some other conventional clinical parameter it may be safe to assume that although we will have a different average value in our experimental group these measures will have a similar variability to that seen in normal animals and so we can obtain measures of variability from existing clinical databases (such as our own hospital records) or previous published studies. If we have performed a pilot study this data will provide the necessary information.

5.2.4 α, β *and power*

The actual possibility of making a type I error is known as α (alpha). If we repeated an experiment 100 times and on 15 occasions we produced a false positive result (we rejected the null hypothesis when it was actually true), the value of α would be 0.15. If we reduce the sample size and when we decrease the effect size we are able to detect and we tend to increase the value of α. Another name for α is the level of statistical significance.

The probability of committing a type II error, i.e. failing to reject the null hypothesis when our alternative hypothesis is actually true, is β (beta). In this case we failed to detect an effect when one was actually present. Were we to repeat an experiment 100 times and on 20 occasions obtained a

false negative result the β value would be 0.2. The value $[1 - \beta]$ is referred to as the power of the experiment, which in this case would be $[1 - 0.2] = 0.8$ or 80%. If β is the probability of not finding a negative result when one actually exists, then the power indicates the probability of finding a difference when one exists. The importance of the value of β or the power of a clinical trial is that it enables us to interpret a negative result. It is unfortunate that there is a tendency not to publish negative results in clinical journals as the absence of a difference of effect between treatments is valuable evidence when making clinical decisions, but perhaps it is even more unfortunate that papers are published reporting no difference between different treatment regimes without an accompanying description of the power of the study, which tells us that the investigators would have been able to demonstrate a difference had there been a difference.

5.2.5   *P value*

When we perform a statistical test on the results from our clinical research we are obtaining an estimate for the α error based on our actual results; this value is referred to as the *P* value.

When the *P* value is less than α (the predetermined level of significance for a difference) it is deemed to be 'non-significant'. This does not necessarily mean that there is no difference (or no association) but that there is a reasonable likelihood that the effect observed may have resulted from chance alone.

Studies typically set thresholds for α at 0.05 and for β at 0.20 (a power of 0.80). This means that if the trial was repeated 100 times on subjects that were not different the reported difference might be expected on five occasions (1 out of every 20) and if the trial was repeated 100 times on subjects that were different the difference would fail to be found on 20 occasions (1:5). It is important to appreciate that these are arbitrary conventions. They represent the minimum standards we should aim for when designing clinical research and deciding on a sample size. We can have considerably more confidence in results that report differences at α levels of 0.01, 0.005 or 0.0001, and those studies that report no difference with β levels of 0.10 or 0.05.

5.2.6 One-sided and two-sided hypotheses

Single- or one-sided hypotheses specify the direction of the difference that is expected or hypothesized whereas a two-sided hypothesis only anticipates that there will be a difference (but that the measure may be either larger or smaller in the experimental group compared to the control group). For example, if we were looking at the effect of a dietary supplement on a group of animals we might hope that it would increase their growth rate compared to a control group. However, should the dietary supplement contain a vast excess in certain vitamins, it might have a toxic effect and lead to impairment of growth. Unless there is a good prior belief that we are expecting an increased growth rate, backed up by strong evidence, we should assume an alternative hypothesis that the experimental group will have a different growth rate but make no assumptions on the direction of the effect.

An example of the appropriate use of a one-sided hypothesis might be used in a study looking at the side effects of the use of prednisolone in the treatment of canine atopy. The mineralocorticoid effects of steroid drugs are well documented and a client is likely to be warned of the likelihood of polyuria and polydipsia. We would not expect the use of prednisolone to result in a decrease in these phenomena and our alternative hypothesis would be that this therapy would increase the incidence when compared to an untreated control group.

When a two-sided or two-tailed (the tails refer to the tails of a distribution curve) statistical test is used the P value that is calculated includes the probabilities of type I errors occurring in each of the two directions, which is approximately twice as likely as when considering errors in one direction. For the majority of statistical tests this means that when they are used to test single-sided hypotheses they generate P values that are approximately half those for a two-sided hypothesis. So a two-sided P value of 0.1 is equivalent to a one-sided P value of 0.05 and the number of subjects required to test a one-sided hypothesis will be considerably lower than the number required to establish statistical significance for a two-sided hypothesis. However, before we start revising our study design it is important to appreciate that we will be unable to test the two-sided hypothesis once we have reduced the numbers. There needs to be a very strong rationale to justify the use of one-sided hypotheses and the assumption of a two-tailed hypothesis builds in a healthy safety margin if we do ultimately use a one-sided statistical test. The adoption of a one-sided hypothesis should never be used only as a means to reduce the sample size.

5.2.7 Multiple hypotheses and post-hoc hypothesis testing

However much we attempt to focus our research we rarely end up with a study that asks a single question or tests a single hypothesis. Because we measure or detect disease using various clinical signs or manifestations, our clinical studies inevitably measure a variety of outcomes. This inevitably complicates the sample size calculations and our plans for statistical analysis.

We conventionally require an α value of 0.05. This means that if we test 20 independent hypotheses in the same experiment the likelihood of obtaining a statistically significant result, purely by chance, is high; in this example it is actually 64% (calculated from $[1 - 0.95^{20}]$). While this may be addressed in the interpretation of results, many statisticians advocate an adjustment in the threshold of statistical significance when multiple hypotheses are being tested.

A strict consideration of multiple hypothesis testing is afforded by applying a Bonferroni correction. This requires that the overall desired level of significance be divided by the number of hypotheses being tested. For example, if we were testing four separate independent hypotheses and would normally use an α value of 0.05 then each individual hypothesis would be tested at an α level of 0.05/4 or 0.00125.

Some authors consider stringent use of the Bonferroni correction to be too limiting to be of practical use in many clinical research scenarios. It is probably of most importance when the likelihood of producing and over-interpreting a false positive result is high. This may occur when the number of hypotheses tested is high and the prior probability of the hypothesis being correct is low; an example of this would be screening a large number of genes for a particular disease association. When the published paper fails to report all the genes that are screened but only emphasizes the associations found, it is important that the researchers follow stringent statistical methodology. On the other hand, clinical studies will be interpreted by readers who can place the results in a clinical context and use pathophysiological reasoning to convert the statistical significance into a clinical significance. Some thought should be given to the appropriate α level to be used. Adjusting α for multiple hypotheses is particularly important when the consequences of a false positive result are substantial, such as falsely concluding that a therapy is effective when this isn't the case.

As has already been suggested it is the likelihood of the hypothesis being correct or the prior probability of its being true that is most important. Browner and Newman (1987) draw an interesting analogy with the use of diagnostic tests.

When you find a modest abnormality in a healthy patient (e.g. an alkaline phophatase level that is 15% greater than the upper limit of normal) you are likely to treat it as a false positive and unlikely to place any clinical significance in the finding. Similarly, a P value of 0.05 in support of

an unlikely hypothesis can be treated with suspicion. Should you encounter an alkaline phosphatase level that is 10 to 20 times greater than normal, although you might consider a laboratory error you are unlikely to believe that it occurred through chance. In the same vein a highly significant P value of 0.001 is unlikely to have occurred through chance although it may be the result of a confounding factor (bias). We are unlikely to ignore extremely abnormal clinical test results and we should not dismiss very low P values as false positives even if the pre-testing possibilities are very low or unlikely.

If we performed 20 tests on a sick cat with polyuria and polydipsia, and found that the only abnormal test result was a highly raised blood urea nitrogen level, we would not dismiss the result because we would expect at least one abnormal result in a panel of this size. We would respond appropriately because the likelihood of this cat having renal failure was already high. When it comes to multiple hypotheses testing there is no reason not to take the same approach. When a carefully reasoned argument is generated by a rational investigator following the accumulation of evidence from a variety of sources, it seems reasonable to assume that there is a high prior probability of the hypothesis being correct even though there is an element of subjective judgement from the investigator.

The results from a study may well turn up some unanticipated associations; we rarely limit ourselves to a single data analysis in a process often referred to as 'data mining' or 'a fishing expedition'. This process may be less cynically referred to as hypothesis generation. Some statistically significant associations may arise that have no logical or rational explanations, while other statistically significant associations may become apparent that do make sense but it just didn't occur to the investigators that these associations would be worth testing for at the planning stage. Both types of association may be of use and are worth reporting. Further investigations may be required to establish the veracity of either type of observation. The important issue is not whether or not the hypothesis was anticipated in the design phase but whether there is a reasonable possibility based on supporting evidence that the hypothesis is true. Where there is no existing evidence to support an unanticipated finding, then that evidence may be a further study designed to test the newly generated hypothesis.

A sound principle is to establish, during the design phase, as many hypotheses as make sense, but to specify one of them as the primary hypothesis, which can be tested statistically without arguments concerning the need for consideration of multiple hypotheses testing. The primary hypothesis provides a focus for the main study objective and a rationale for the main sample size calculation.

5.3 Testing for statistical significance

There are two basic statistical tests that every clinical researcher should be able to use; these are the chi-squared test and the Student's *t* test. Anyone with high school mathematical skills can perform them, and they are part of the standard library of functions that are available in almost all spreadsheet programs.

5.3.1 The chi-squared test

The chi-squared test is used to compare the proportion of subjects in each of two groups having one of two outcomes (dichotomous outcomes). A clinical example would be a test of antibiotic use in the treatment of kennel cough. Dogs could be given antibiotics or a placebo, and the outcome measure might be that they are cured or they continue to cough on the fifth day after treatment.

The chi-squared test is always two-sided although there is an equivalent for a one-sided hypothesis called the *Z* test.

5.3.2 The Student's *t* test

The Student's *t* test, sometimes just referred to as the *t* test, is used to compare the difference between the mean of a continuous outcome (interval data) derived from one group with the mean from another group. A simple veterinary example could be comparing the mean growth rate of a group of animals receiving one diet with the mean growth rate from a group on another diet. The *t* test assumes that the parameter being measured has a distribution that approximates to a normal distribution (it produces a bell-shaped curve where the mean, mode and median values are roughly the same). Fortunately, use of the *t* test is valid for many different distributions. The *t* test only really falls down when there are fewer than 30 subjects or if there is a small number of very high and/or very low values.

The *t* test can be performed as either a one-tailed test to test a one-sided hypothesis or as a two-tailed test to test a two-sided hypothesis.

5.3.3 Establishing correlation

In a study that was investigating the value of looking at antibodies in milk an obvious experiment would be to take serum and milk samples from a group of dairy cows and compare the results of an antibody test conducted on the two samples. We would not expect the milk and serum results from an individual cow to be identical but we would expect them to correlate; in other words if a cow had a high serum level of antibodies we would expect a high milk level of antibodies when compared to the milk levels in other cows.

If we were to plot a graph of the milk results on the *y*-axis and the serum results on the *x*-axis, we would expect the individual results to cluster about a line with a positive gradient that intercepts the *x*- or *y*-axis somewhere near the origin of the graph. If there was poor correlation we might see a similar pattern but would expect an increasing number of results that were some distance from this line, and it would be more difficult to determine the best place to put the line.

The correlation coefficient (*r*) is a measure of the strength of linear association (how closely the result fits the line). It varies from +1 to −1, with negative values indicating that the line has a negative gradient (i.e. if one parameter of a result is high, the other parameter will be low). The closer the absolute value of *r* is to 1, the closer the results cluster around the line and the more perfect the correlation between the two measures is. Realistically we can't expect to obtain a perfect correlation but something like the correlation between height and weight within a breed would give a correlation coefficient of around 0.9. The proportion of the observed variability accounted for by the association can be derived from the square of *r*; thus a correlation producing an *r* of 0.6 indicates that 0.36 (0.6 × 0.6) of the variation in one measure is accounted for by the value of the other measure (and vice versa).

When the data being compared are continuous interval data, as in the example above, then the test used and the calculation performed are for Pearson's correlation coefficient. When the data are ranked ordinal values then Spearman's ranked correlation coefficient is required. (It is worth noting that antibody measurements producing an absolute measure of quantity (say in ng/ml) are continuous data while antibody measurements reported as titres should be treated as ordinal data.)

5.4   Other statistical tests and choosing the appropriate statistical test

While life would be easy if all our statistical needs were addressed by just a handful of widely applicable tests, we have to face reality and acknowledge that the reason that there is an entire discipline devoted to unravelling our statistical conundrums is that life isn't easy. It is beyond the scope of this textbook to provide an exhaustive description of all the available tests.

As a general principle parametric statistical tests (those performed on continuous variables) are more powerful than non-parametric tests (those performed on ordinal or nominal variables). More 'powerful' tests are more sensitive and normally require fewer subjects to achieve statistical significance.

Each test that has been designed will only provide a valid *P* value if the data that are fed into it adhere to some rules and/or assumptions. For example, the *t* test described above requires continuous values which have a roughly normal distribution. In order to work out which test may be appropriate we need to understand some of the properties of our data.

5.4.1   *What type of data are being collected?*

Are they nominal, ordinal or interval? Nominal data are categories without ranking such as breed, sex or blood group. Ordinal data are categories that are ranked. Clinical signs such as exercise intolerance might be described as slight, minor, moderate or extreme. The categories indicate magnitude but not on a necessarily uniform scale. Interval data describe continuous values that are measured on a uniform scale such as temperature, leucocyte counts and hormone levels.

5.4.2   *How many groups are being compared?*

Do we have a single group, two groups or more than two groups? If we are looking at the same group but at different time points they represent two groups.

5.4.3   *Are the groups independent or related?*

If the selection of an individual in one group has no influence on the selection of an individual in

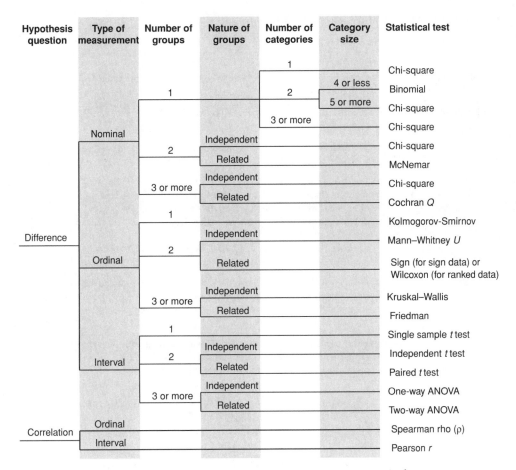

Figure 5.2 A simplified decision tree for choosing the appropriate statistical test.

another group then they are independent. An example of independent groups would be the treatment groups in a randomized controlled trial. An example of related groups would be when we use the group of animals as their own controls in a study involving repeated measures before and after treatment. Another example would be the pairing of cases and controls in a case-control study; here the animals might be matched on age, breed and sex.

5.4.4   What is the number of categories?

This only concerns nominal data. If our categories were based on sex we might use four categories:

entire male, entire female, neutered male and neutered female.

5.4.5   How large are the categories?

Again this is only relevant to nominal data and we need to know how many animals there are in each category.

5.4.6   Choosing the test

When the answers to the questions above are known the decision tree shown in Fig. 5.2 can be used to indicate the appropriate test. A summary of the commonly used tests is given in Table 5.1.

Table 5.1   Summary of the statistical tests listed in Fig. 5.2.

Test	Description
Parametric tests	
Single sample *t* test	Single-sample Student's *t* test used to compare the sample mean with a hypothesized mean
Independent *t* test	Student's independent *t* test used to compare the means of two independent sets of measurements
Paired *t* test	Student's paired *t* test used to compare the means of two sets of measurements when the samples are paired (e.g. two sets of measurements from the same group of animals taken on different occasions)
One-way analysis of variance (ANOVA)	Sometimes called an *F* test, this is closely related to the *t* test but the major difference is that whereas the *t* test measures the difference between the means of two groups, an ANOVA tests the difference between the means of two or more groups A one-way ANOVA, or single factor ANOVA, tests differences between groups that are only classified on one independent variable (e.g. age or sex, but not both)
Two-way analysis of variance	Two-way ANOVA (also called factorial ANOVA) is used to examine the effect of more than one factor at the same time (e.g. the effect on the growth rate of pigs when fed diets containing different salt concentrations, and different amounts of crude fibre)
Pearson *r*	This test produces a correlation coefficient (*r*) for parametric data The value of *r* ranges from −1 to 1 where 0 represents no correlation, 1 indicates perfect correlation and −1 indicates an inverse correlation
Nonparametric tests	
Binomial test	This is a statistical test referring to a binary process such as would be expected to generate outcomes with a binomial distribution A value for the expected proportion is hypothesized and the difference of the actual value from this is assessed as a value of alpha
Chi-squared test	Pearson's chi-squared test, also known as the chi-squared goodness-of-fit test, which is used to test the distribution of individuals to an expected series of categories (e.g. are road traffic accidents equally distributed over the 12 months of the year?) In a two-by-two contingency table, when numbers are small (sum of counts is less than 100), Fisher's exact test should be used
McNemar test	The McNemar test is a test on a two-by-two contingency table when the two classification factors are dependent or when you want to test the difference between paired proportions, e.g. in studies in which patients serve as their own control or in studies with 'before and after' design
Cochran *Q* test (McNemar on repeated measures)	Cochran's *Q* test is used on replicated measurements data with binary responses. It tests a difference in effects among two or more treatments applied to the same set of experimental units
Kolmogorov–Smirnov test	For a single sample of data, the Kolmogorov–Smirnov test is used to test whether or not the sample of data is consistent with a specified distribution function (it can also be used to determine if two datasets differ significantly) The Kolmogorov–Smirnov test has the advantage of making no assumption about the distribution of data (it is non-parametric and distribution free) It is less sensitive than equivalent parametric tests such as the *t* test

(*cont.*)

Table 5.1 *(cont.)*

Test	Description
Mann–Whitney U test	The Mann–Whitney U test is a non-parametric statistical significance test for assessing whether or not the difference in medians between two samples of observations is statistically significant The null hypothesis is that the two samples are drawn from a single population and therefore that the medians are equal. It requires the two samples to be independently measured, at least at an ordinal level, i.e. we can at least say, of any two observations, which is the greater It is one of the best-known non-parametric significance tests. It is sometimes also called the Mann–Whitney–Wilcoxon (MWW) test or the Wilcoxon rank-sum test
Sign test	The sign test is designed to test a hypothesis about the location of a population distribution. It is most often used to test the hypothesis about a population median and often involves the use of matched pairs, for example, before and after data, in which case it tests for a median difference of zero The sign test does not require the assumption that the population is normally distributed. In many applications, this test is used in place of the one sample t test when the normality assumption is questionable It is a less powerful alternative to the Wilcoxon signed ranks test, but does not assume that the population probability distribution is symmetric This test can also be applied when the observations in a sample of data are ranks, that is ordinal data rather than direct measurements
Wilcoxon Mann–Whitney test	The Wilcoxon Mann–Whitney test is one of the most powerful of the non-parametric tests for comparing two populations. It is used to test the null hypothesis that two populations have identical distribution functions against the alternative hypothesis that the two distribution functions differ only with respect to location (median), if at all The Wilcoxon Mann–Whitney test does not require the assumption that the differences between the two samples are normally distributed. In many applications, the Wilcoxon Mann–Whitney test is used in place of the two sample t test when the normality assumption is questionable This test can also be applied when the observations in a sample of data are ranks, that is ordinal data rather than direct measurements
Kruskal–Wallis test	The Kruskal–Wallis test is a non-parametric test used to compare three or more samples. It is used to test the null hypothesis that all populations have identical distribution functions against the alternative hypothesis that at least two of the samples differ only with respect to location (median), if at all. It is the analogue to the F-test used in analysis of variance. While analysis of variance tests depend on the assumption that all populations under comparison are normally distributed, the Kruskal-Wallis test places no such restriction on the comparison. It is a logical extension of the Wilcoxon-Mann-Whitney test
Friedman test	The Friedman test is a non-parametric test to compare three or more matched groups. It is also called Friedman two-way analysis of variance by ranks (because repeated measures one-way ANOVA is the same as two-way ANOVA without any replicates) The P value answers this question: If the median difference really is zero, what is the chance that random sampling would result in a median difference as far from zero (or more so) as observed in this experiment?
Spearman rho (ρ)	This test produces a correlation coefficient (r) for non-parametric data. The value of r ranges from -1 to 1 where 0 represents no correlation, 1 indicates perfect correlation and -1 indicates an inverse correlation

Statistical tests that use interval data or continuous variables are described as parametric tests. Parametric tests are more powerful than non-parametric tests (i.e. they have a higher probability of rejecting the null hypothesis when the alternative hypothesis is true). If we can use interval data (continuous variables) then we should. The requirements for the use of parametric tests are:

- The subjects in the groups are randomly selected from the population.
- Measurements are interval data (continuous variables).
- The data are normally distributed.
- The variances (the spread of the values) in the groups are equal.

When any one of these conditions is not met we have to use a non-parametric test. If you have parametric data, don't immediately despair if you believe that your data fail to match the criteria needed for a parametric test but consult with your statistician over your data; their greater depth of knowledge and experience will enable them to help you make the right decision. If you do have to use a non-parametric test you will have to convert your interval data into ranked ordinal data.

Further information on all the statistical tests mentioned in this chapter can be found in any good statistical textbook. In the further reading section at the end of this chapter are some sources that the authors have found useful.

5.5   Reference

Browner WS, Newman TB (1987) Are all significant *P* values created equal? The analogy between diagnostic tests and clinical research. *JAMA* **257**: 2459–63.

5.6   Further reading

Dohoo I, Martin W, Stryhn H (2003) *Veterinary Epidemiologic Research*, AVC Inc., Charlottestown, Prince Edward Island.

Hulley SB, Cummings SR, Browner WS, Grady DG, Newman TB (2007) Getting ready to estimate sample size: Hypotheses and underlying principles. In *Designing Clinical Research*, 3rd edn, Lippincott Williams and Wilkins, Philadelphia, pp 51–63.

Pocock SJ (1983) Basic principles of statistical analysis. In *Clinical Trials: A Practical Approach*, John Wiley and Sons, Chichester, pp 176–86.

Smith RD (2005) Statistical significance. In *Veterinary Clinical Epidemiology*, CRC/Taylor & Francis, Boca Raton, pp 137–62.

Thrusfield, M. (2005) Demonstrating association. In: *Veterinary Epidemiology*, 3rd edn, Blackwell Publishing, Oxford, pp 247–65.

Woodward M (2005) *Epidemiology: Study Design and Data Analysis*, 2nd edn, Chapman & Hall/CRC, London.

5.7   MCQs

1 *What is a type I error?*

  (a)   A false positive result.
  (b)   A false negative result.

2 *What is a type II error?*

  (a)   A false positive result.
  (b)   A false negative result.

3 *What test should be used to compare the means of two sets of measurements when the samples are paired (e.g. two sets of measurements from the same group of animals taken on different occasions)?*

  (a)   Student's *t* test.
  (b)   Chi-squared test.
  (c)   One-way analysis of variance.
  (d)   Pearson *r* calculation.
  (e)   Mann–Whitney *U* test.

4 *What test is used to test the distribution of individuals to an expected series of categories (e.g. are road traffic accidents equally distributed in the 12 months of the year)?*

  (a)   Student's *t* test.
  (b)   Chi-squared test.
  (c)   One-way analysis of variance.
  (d)   Pearson *r* calculation.
  (e)   Mann–Whitney *U* test.

5 *What is a correlation coefficient a measure of?*

(a) The variability of a measure.
(b) The strength of linear association.
(c) A type II error.
(d) Statistical power.
(e) The intervals between data.

6 *What does β (the beta value) represent?*

(a) The probability of making a type I error.
(b) The probability of making a type II error.
(c) The probability of obtaining a false positive result.
(d) The probability of obtaining a false negative result.
(e) The probability of the result being wrong (either false negative or false positive).

7 *What criteria have to be satisfied for groups to be 'independent'?*

(a) That animals in a group are from different locations.
(b) That animals are selected from different populations.
(c) That animals are matched only in some regards but not for the outcome variable of interest.
(d) That the selection of an individual has no influence on the selection of an individual in another group.
(e) That the selection of an individual is performed by pairing on a single selection criterion.

8 *How can the variance be estimated in advance of collecting the study data?*

(a) Using historical data from the same or a similar population.

(b) Using a variance value from results published in a similar study.
(c) By performing a pilot study.
(d) By estimating on pathophysiological principles from laboratory data.
(e) By seeking advice from colleagues or laboratories that have experience of measuring the variable of interest.

9 *When a P value is reported as <0.05 what does this mean?*

(a) That there is a 5% or less chance of obtaining a false negative result.
(b) That there is a 95% or more chance of obtaining a false negative result.
(c) That there is a 5% or less chance of obtaining a false positive result.
(d) That there is a 95% or more chance of obtaining a false positive result.
(e) That the value of β (beta) is 5% or less.

10 *What adjustment should be made when testing multiple hypotheses from the same data set?*

(a) A chi-squared test adjustment.
(b) A *Z* adjustment.
(c) A Pearson adjustment.
(d) A Bonferroni adjustment.
(e) Dividing the desired overall *P* value threshold by the number of hypotheses being tested to provide a new threshold for the *P* value for the individual tests.

5.8 MCQ answers

1 (a); 2 (b); 3 (a); 4 (b); 5 (b) and (d); 6 (d); 7 (d); 8 Any of the answers could provide the basis for a rational estimate of variability for a measure; 9 (c); 10 (d) and (e) (which is a description of the Bonferonni adjustment).

6

HOW MANY ANIMALS/ PATIENTS ARE NEEDED? ESTIMATING THE SAMPLE SIZE

Objectives

After reading this chapter readers should:

- appreciate the importance of statistical advice at the planning stage
- be able to estimate sample size and power
- understand some basic statistical tests.

6.1   Introduction

Having introduced the basic principles behind sample size estimates we are now ready to consider actually making the sample size or power calculation for our own study. Books such as this always fall between pillar and post for the individual user. The authors make a valiant attempt to provide some theoretical background so readers understand the basic principles and terminology, and then provide a range of examples that cover the main study design types. It is hoped that the examples or recipes are suitably generic and that the reader can then just replace the parameter values with those appropriate to their own studies and arrive at an easy answer. Sadly, the real world is not like that. Inevitably, much to the reader's frustration, their own study design fails to mirror one of the examples. It is important to appreciate that a basic textbook such as this is not designed to replace or be a substitute for the expertise of a statistician or epidemiologist with clinical research experience. When large research projects are undertaken or we are forced to use complex study designs it is imperative that we seek their advice. However, we can gain maximum benefit from their input when we have some basic knowledge and can predict the information they will need in order to assist us. Think hard about your study design and return to your research question: Have you chosen the simplest design to answer your primary hypothesis? Is your output measure the best one to test your hypothesis? You may find that changes to your study design that add work or expense to the collection of better quality data will be well rewarded by decreased work and complexity in the analysis phase, and lead to better answers

to your question. The sayings 'garbage in leads to garbage out' and 'you can't make a silk purse out of a sow's ear' are both applicable to clinical research. Although statisticians will always do their best to help you achieve a 'significant result', what we really want to achieve is a clear, true answer to your research question.

6.2   Producing the sample size estimate

The groundwork for undertaking the sample size estimation is described in the previous chapter. There are several variations on the procedures required to perform the sample size or power calculation but they all have the following steps in common:

1. State the null hypothesis and either a one- or two-tailed alternative hypothesis.
2. Determine the appropriate statistical approach or test.
   - (a) Comparison of two means
   - (b) Comparing two proportions
   - (c) Correlation coefficient
   - (d) Descriptive study of a continuous variable
   - (e) Descriptive study of a proportion
   - (f) Other (seek specialist statistical advice)
3. Choose a clinically significant effect size (i.e. the difference between the mean values or the proportions of the control and experimental groups with the outcome of interest).
4. Make an estimate of the variation (standard deviation) of the effect variable (when a parametric test is to be used).
5. Select error thresholds for α and β (often used values are 0.05 and 0.1 respectively for a 5% probability of a false positive result and a 10% probability of a false negative result – a power of 90%).

6.2.1   *Estimating the variance or standard deviation*

An estimate of the sample variance is required when a study is comparing the means of a measurement between two groups and it may be difficult to obtain. The best option is to obtain some pilot data or a sample of data from the population that is going to be providing the subjects. Sometimes this can be obtained from hospital records. There may be reports from similar studies in the literature that suggest an appropriate figure.

Variability is often reported as either the standard deviation (SD or σ) or as the standard error of the mean (SEM). For the purposes of sample size calculation the standard deviation is the more useful figure. Statisticians may prefer to use the variance, which is the square of the SD. It is relatively easy to convert between the various measures:

$$SD = SEM \times \sqrt{N}$$

where N is the number of subjects that make up the mean.

Confidence intervals (CIs) are increasingly used in clinical journals to indicate the clinically significant range of a mean (or a value). If the mean is not reported (i.e. a range is given), then the mean can be obtained by adding the upper and lower limits together and dividing by two.

An estimate of the standard deviation from a confidence interval range is:

$$SD = \frac{\text{upper CI level} \times \text{mean}}{1.96} \times \sqrt{N}$$

6.2.2   Deciding on an effect size

The effect size is the smallest difference between the study groups that the investigator wishes to be able to detect and achieve statistical significance. Obviously the smaller the difference you want to detect, the larger the number of subjects that will be required. Clinical research should aim to inform clinical practice and so effect size targets should be set to a level that would be of

interest to a clinician. Very small effect sizes may require large numbers, and while they will provide statistical significance to relatively small differences this may be of little relevance to clinical practice.

For a study looking at proportions (e.g. outcomes that are described as 'successes' or 'failures') the difference in proportions is likely to be of clinical interest (e.g. as clinicians we might be interested in a new treatment that had a 10% or greater success rate as compared to an existing treatment) but for the purposes of the sample size calculation we need to have an estimate for the baseline proportion in our control group. This is because the sample size needed to detect a 10% better success rate compared to a control group with a 50% success rate is greater than a 10% better success rate compared to a control group with an 80% success rate.

6.3   Sample size required per group for the comparison of two means

This calculation will produce an estimate for the size of the two groups required to compare the means of continuous variables analysed using a t test. Sample size calculators are found in a variety of statistical computer packages and can be readily found on the internet.

Pocock (1983) describes a relatively simple calculation that can easily be implemented in a spreadsheet document:

$$n = \frac{2\sigma^2}{\delta^2} \times f(\alpha, \beta)$$

where n is the sample size required for each group (the answer we are seeking), δ is the magnitude of the difference between the means of the measurements in the two groups (the effect size), σ is the standard deviation of the measurement and $f(\alpha, \beta)$ is a function of the chosen α and β thresholds (values for these are given in

Table 6.1   Values for f(α,β) for different error thresholds.

α value (type I error)	β (type II error)			
	0.05	0.1	0.2	0.5
0.10	10.8	8.6	6.2	2.7
0.05	13.0	10.5	7.9	3.8
0.02	15.8	13.0	10	5.4
0.01	17.8	14.9	11.7	6.6

Table 6.1). From this formula it is evident that larger effect sizes and lower variabilities will reduce the sample size, which accords with our expectations.

This is a relatively simple approach to the sample size calculation and there are more rigorous approaches to calculation that may provide a better estimate for studies using particular variations of the *t* test or when the sample size is small. It can be a little bewildering for inexperienced researchers to discover a variety of different sample size calculators or formulae all giving different answers to what seems to be the same question. There tend to be relatively minor differences with the larger sample sizes although the proportional differences at the other end of the scale (often where veterinary clinical studies lie) may be important. An alternative method of obtaining a sample size estimate for comparing means is given in Appendix 6.2. This table uses the *t* statistic and provides a slightly more robust estimate for studies with sample sizes with fewer than 30 in each group.

6.4   Sample size required per group for the comparison of multiple means

While the sample size is best calculated to consider the answering of a single focused clinical question, there are occasions when multiple comparisons may form part of the main study question.

The statistical method required for analysis is the analysis of variance (ANOVA).

6.5   Sample size required per group for the comparison of two proportions

In many veterinary clinical research situations the outcome of most interest is dichotomous, e.g. following an intervention the outcome may be either a 'success' or a 'failure' for the patient.

Pocock (1983) describes a relatively simple calculation for the sample size required for the comparison of two proportions that can easily be implemented using a spreadsheet program:

$$n = \frac{p_1 \times (100 - p_1) + p_2 \times (100 - p_2)}{(p_2 - p_1)^2} \times f(\alpha, \beta)$$

where *n* is the sample size required for each group (the answer we are seeking), p_1 is the proportion of the outcome in the first of the groups as a percentage, p_2 is the proportion of the outcome in the second of the groups as a percentage, f (α, β) is a function of the chosen α and β thresholds (values are given in Table 6.1; this is the same function used for the sample size calculation for the comparison of two means).

From the formula it can be seen that sample size is proportional to the inverse of the square of the difference in proportions and so discriminating between larger differences of proportions will require a smaller number of subjects.

This formula provides the number required for each group; when more than one group is being compared to a control then the same group size can be used for each of the additional experimental groups.

As for the previous calculation of sample size when comparing two means, this calculation ignores corrections that are required when one of the group's proportions is very small (i.e. less than 10%), which may lead to an underestimate of the sample size. A table with corrected sample size estimates for this situation is given in Appendix 6.1.

6.5.1 Power calculations – what to do when the sample size is fixed

The power of a study is $1-\beta$, the probability of not obtaining a false negative result. When a statistically significant result (e.g. a result with $P > 0.05$) is achieved once a study has been completed, the pre-study estimate of the power is largely irrelevant. However, if no statistically significant result is achieved the question arises 'Is this negative result a false negative?' This question can only be answered if the power of the study is known. A post-hoc calculation of the power provides evidence for the statistical significance of a negative result.

Sometimes clinical researchers have little choice about the number of subjects that are available. This may be the situation in a retrospective study or where the study design dictates that there is a limited source of subjects. In this case the sample size calculation formulae can be used to obtain an estimate of the maximum effect size that is likely to be statistically significant. While lesser effect sizes may be clinically interesting at least a judgement can be made about the value of the research and this may help to justify the study to a funding body.

6.5.2 Example: calculating a sample size for a Student's t test

A study is being designed to investigate the effect of neutering on aggressive behaviour in bitches. A previous behavioural study has described a scoring system that measures aggressive behaviour on a scale of 0 (no signs of aggression) to 8 (extreme aggressive behaviour). The scale is based on objective behavioural observations and non-integer values result from the mean values from multiple observations. The result from the previous study performed on entire bitches reported a mean value of 4.1 with 95% of bitches in the range 1.6 to 6.6. The distribution of aggression scores indicated an approximately normal distribution (the mean, median and mode have the same value and the curve has a symmetrical bell-shaped appearance).

We wish to be able to detect a difference of 0.5 of an aggression unit. We want our study to have a power of 90% (i.e. the probability of detecting a true negative result) and a P value of 0.05 for our positive result.

We don't have a value for the standard deviation but for a normal distribution 95% of the values would fall between the mean ± 2 SD; using the previous study we can estimate the standard deviation as:

$$SD = (6.6 - 1.6)/4 = 1.25$$

It is possible that neutering may increase or decrease aggression and so we will be testing a two-tailed hypothesis.

Using the calculation described in section 6.3:

$$n = \frac{2\sigma^2}{\delta^2} \times f(\alpha, \beta)$$

$n = \dfrac{2 \times 1.25^2}{0.5^2} \times 10.5$ (using Table 6.1 for the value of $f(\alpha, \beta)$ for $\alpha = 0.05$ and $\beta = 0.1$)

$$n = 131.25 \approx 131$$

If we use the tables in Appendix 6.2 we need to choose Table 6.A2(b) for $\alpha = 0.05$: the standardized effect size is:

$$E/SD = 0.5/1.25 = 0.4$$

From the E/SD row for 0.4, we can read off the sample size for a β value of 0.1 as 133. This is a slightly larger sample size due to the greater accuracy of the table. For our study we decide on 150 bitches per group to allow for some dropout of recruited animals.

6.5.3 Example: calculating a sample size for a chi-squared test

A study is interested in looking at the ability of a vaccine to reduce respiratory disease in housed calves. The current risk of respiratory disease in the farms that have been recruited for the study is 20%. A decrease in the risk of disease of 5% or greater is of clinical interest. We want our study to have a power of 80% and we will be using a value for α of 0.05. The study will compare a group of calves vaccinated before being introduced to the calf house with a group of unvaccinated calves.

Using the formula in section 6.5:

$$n = \frac{p_1 \times (100 - p_1) + p_2 \times (100 - p_2)}{(p_2 - p_1)^2} \times f(\alpha, \beta)$$

$$n = \frac{15 \times (100 - 15) + 20 \times (100 - 20)}{(20 - 15)^2}$$

$$\times 7.9$$

(using Table 6.1 for the value of f (α, β) for α = 0.05 and β = 0.2)

$n = 908.5 \approx 909$ (animals per group)

Using the tables in Appendix 6.1, we need to choose Table 6.A1(b) α = 0.05 and β = 0.02: the smallest proportion would be 0.2 − 0.05 = 0.15 and the difference would be 0.05; reading from the table this will give us a sample size of 944 animals per group. This is higher than the calculated value due to the assumptions that are used to simplify the formula. A sample size of 950 is chosen to allow for withdrawals.

6.6 Sample size techniques for analytic studies and experiments

Although the process for calculating a sample size will vary according to the study design the basic process is as follows:

1. Determine the null hypothesis, which should include whether it is one-sided or two-sided.
2. Select the most appropriate statistical test based on the predictor variable and the output variable.
3. Make a decision on the minimum effect size that the study should be able to detect. For

a descriptive study of a single value this may include the confidence interval (the likely range of values) and the confidence level (the probability that the found value lies in this range). A 95% confidence interval is often used.

4. Where appropriate (i.e. necessary) estimate the variability of the output measure.
5. Where appropriate make a decision on the appropriate α and β levels (an α of 0.05 and β of 0.2 are the minimum conventional values for most experiments).
6. Use the appropriate table or formula to estimate the sample size.
   (a) Sample size when a study aims to measure the value of a proportion (a dichotomous variable). Tables may be found in Appendix 6.3.
   (b) Sample size when a study aims to measure the value of a continuous variable. Tables may be found in Appendix 6.4.
   (c) Sample size when a study aims to test whether a correlation coefficient differs from zero. Tables may be found in Appendix 6.5.

6.7 Further considerations when estimating sample size

6.7.1 Missing data

It is likely that in any clinical research project there will be unanticipated loss of subjects at some stage. Pets may be involved in road traffic accidents, clients may move home and farm animals may be sold or culled. These dropouts should be allowed for in the initial study design. When reviewing scientific papers referees will be extremely suspicious if an author reports more than 20% dropouts as there will always be the suspicion that they may represent a significant population that would have influenced the result of the study. In any event it would be wise to allow for somewhere between 10 and 20% dropouts when making the sample estimate.

6.7.2   Survival analysis

Oncology studies and research on the therapy of severe disease may look at survival as an outcome for the subjects involved. Although the outcome variable, say the number of days, weeks or months, may seem to be a continuous variable, the t test is not appropriate. The data are not normally distributed, but more pertinently the actual outcome of interest is the proportion of animals that are still alive at each time point. For the purpose of providing a sample estimate a reasonable approximation can be made by dichotomizing the outcome variable at the end of the anticipated follow-up period (e.g. the proportion surviving for 300 days and longer) and using a chi-squared sample size estimation.

6.7.3   Clustering of samples

It is sometimes necessary to investigate subjects that are clustered in groups. An obvious example is looking at subjects from veterinary practices. Say we wanted to investigate the effect of continuing education on the prescribing habits of veterinary practitioners. One group of practices would receive the education and a second group of practices would act as a control. The outcome measure would be obtained by randomly sampling the client records. Is the sample size the number of practices (e.g. 10 practices) or the number of client records (e.g. 20 clients from each practice, a total of 200)? The answer is somewhere between the two and will depend on the distribution of the outcome measure both within the practice and between the practices. Obtaining a sample estimate may require some pilot data and in any event the study design would benefit from the assistance of a statistician.

6.7.4   Categorized data

When ordinal data are used (data that are ranked on a non-uniform scale) it may be possible to treat these as continuous data for the purposes of sample size estimation. If the number of categories is relatively high (more than six) and if

averaging them is not irrational, this is a legitimate approach.

6.8   Reference

Pocock SJ (1983) The size of a clinical trial. In: *Clinical Trials: A Practical Approach*. John Wiley and Sons, Chichester, pp 123–141.

6.9   Further reading

Dohoo I, Martin W, Stryhn H (2003) Sampling (section 2.10). In: *Veterinary Epidemiologic Research*, AVC Inc., Charlottestown, Prince Edward Island, pp 39–49.

Friedman LM, Furberg CD, DeMets DL (1998) Sample size. In: *Fundamentals of Clinical Trials*, 3rd edn, Springer-Verlag, New York, pp 94–129.

Hulley SB, Cummings SR, Browner WS, Grady DG, Newman TB (2007) Estimating sample size and power. In: *Designing Clinical Research*, 3rd edn, Lippincott Williams and Wilkins, Philadelphia, pp 65–93.

Pocock SJ (1983) The size of a clinical trial. In: *Clinical Trials: A Practical Approach*, John Wiley and Sons, Chichester, pp 123–141.

Woodward M (2005) Sample size determination. In: *Epidemiology: Study Design and Data Analysis*, 2nd edn, Chapman & Hall/CRC, London, pp 381–426.

6.10   MCQs

1   *What is meant by the power of a study?*

(a)   The probability that the test will not produce a false positive result.

(b)   The likelihood that the correct number of samples has been included in a study.

(c)   The probability that the study will produce a true positive result.

(d)   The probability that the study will produce a false negative result.

(e)   The probability that the study will NOT produce a false negative result.

2   *What value for α equates to a P value of 0.01?*

(a) $\alpha = 0.99$

(b) $\alpha = 0.01$

(c) $\alpha = 99$

(d) $\alpha = 1$

(e) $\alpha = 99\%$

3 *What is meant by a two-tailed hypothesis?*

(a) A two-tailed hypothesis is one that tests two hypotheses.
(b) A two-tailed hypothesis accepts that a difference may be due to either an increase or a decrease in the value measured in the experimental group compared to the control group.
(c) A two-tailed hypothesis accepts that a difference may only be due to an increase in the value measured in the experimental group compared to the control group.
(d) A two-tailed hypothesis accepts that a difference may only be due to a decrease in the value measured in the experimental group compared to the control group.
(e) A two-tailed hypothesis is one that suggests that there is no difference between the two groups.

4 *What is the relationship between sample size calculations for one-tailed and two-tailed hypotheses?*

(a) The sample for a one-tailed test is half that for a two-tailed test.
(b) The sample for a one-tailed test is twice that for a two-tailed test.
(c) The sample size for a one-tailed test at a particular α level is the same as for a two-tailed test at twice that α level.
(d) The sample size for a one-tailed test at a particular α level is the same as for a two-tailed test at half that α level.
(e) There is no relationship between sample size calculations for one-tailed and two-tailed tests.

5 *What statistical analysis is used for comparing multiple means from more than one group?*

(a) Mann–Whitney U test.
(b) Analysis of variance (ANOVA).
(c) Student's t test.
(d) Bonferroni test.
(e) Chi-squared test.

6 *What is the definition of a 95% confidence interval?*

(a) That there is a 5% probability that the result is a false positive.

(b) That there is a 95% probability of a false negative result.
(c) That there is a 95% probability that the mean answer is correct.
(d) That there is a 5% probability that a repeat of the trial would produce an answer within the confidence intervals.
(e) That there is a 95% probability that a repeat of the trial would produce an answer within the confidence intervals.

7 *What information is required to calculate the sample size for a study comparing the means of a measure from two groups?*

(a) The variance of the measure.
(b) The standard deviation of the measure.
(c) The minimum difference between the two means that the study hopes to detect.
(d) A decision on the desired α value.
(e) A decision on the desired β value.

8 *What information is required to calculate the sample size for a study comparing the proportions from a dichotomous measure from two groups?*

(a) The variance of the measure.
(b) The standard deviation of the measure.
(c) The two proportions that represent the minimum effect size to be identified.
(d) A decision on the desired α value.
(e) A decision on the desired β value.

9 *Which of the following is the correct formula for deriving the standard deviation (SD) from a standard error of the mean (SEM) where N is the number of subjects that make up the mean?*

(a) $SEM = SD \times \sqrt{N}$
(b) $SD = SEM \times \sqrt{N}$
(c) $SD = N \times \sqrt{SEM}$
(d) $SD = SEM \times N^2$
(e) $SD = SEM \times N$

10 *What is the value of a power calculation performed after a study has been performed?*

(a) A study result is not statistically significant in the absence of a power calculation.

(b)   Journal editors will not accept a paper for publication without a power calculation.

(c)   A positive result is not statistically significant in the absence of a power calculation.

(d)   A power calculation provides evidence that a negative result is unlikely to be a false negative result.

(e)   There is no value in a post-hoc power calculation.

6.11   MCQ answers

1 (e) The power of a study is $(1 - \beta)$. This is the probability that the study will not produce a false negative result (β is the probability of a false negative result).

2 (b); 3 (b) The answers (c) and (d) describe one-tailed hypotheses; 4 (c); 5 (b); 6 (e); 7 (a) or (b), (c), (d) and (e). The standard deviation and variance can be derived from each other; 8 (c), (d) and (e); 9 (b); 10 (d)

Appendix 6.1: Tables estimating sample size group for comparing two proportions

First choose the appropriate table. Tables 6.A1(a), 6.A1(b) and 6.A1(c) are for sample sizes for proportions 0.05–0.90 for the smallest proportion and a difference of 0.05–0.50; Tables 6.A1(d), 6.A1(e) and 6.A1(f) are for sample sizes for proportions 0.01–0.10 for the smallest proportion and a difference of 0.01–0.10.

There are three tables for each set of proportions, providing sample sizes for different combinations of α and β values. Choose a table with your chosen error thresholds.

Having selected the two proportions that the study should be able to discriminate, take the lower proportion (least P) and find the value from the left-hand column to identify the correct row. Use the value of the other proportion to select a column and read the required group size from the intersection of the selected row and column.

Table 6.A1(a) Sample size group for comparing two proportions (0.05–0.90 and 0.05–0.50) for a two-tailed hypothesis for $\alpha = 0.10$ and $\beta = 0.20$.

Least P	Difference between P_1 and P_2									
	0.05	0.10	0.15	0.20	0.25	0.30	0.35	0.40	0.45	0.50
0.05	381	129	72	47	35	27	22	18	15	13
0.10	578	175	91	58	41	31	24	20	16	14
0.15	751	217	108	67	46	34	26	21	17	15
0.20	900	251	121	74	50	36	28	22	18	15
0.25	1024	278	132	79	53	38	29	23	18	15
0.30	1123	300	141	83	55	39	29	23	18	15
0.35	1197	315	146	85	56	39	29	23	18	15
0.40	1246	325	149	86	56	39	29	22	17	14
0.45	1271	328	149	85	55	38	28	21	16	13
0.50	1271	325	146	83	53	36	26	20	15	—
0.55	1246	315	141	79	50	34	24	18	—	—
0.60	1197	300	132	74	46	31	22	—	—	—
0.65	1123	278	121	67	41	27	—	—	—	—
0.70	1024	251	108	58	35	—	—	—	—	—
0.75	900	217	91	47	—	—	—	—	—	—
0.80	751	175	72	—	—	—	—	—	—	—
0.85	578	129	—	—	—	—	—	—	—	—
0.90	381	—	—	—	—	—	—	—	—	—

Table 6.A1(b)   Sample size group for comparing two proportions (0.05–0.90 and 0.05–0.50) for a two-tailed hypothesis for $\alpha = 0.05$ and $\beta = 0.20$.

Least P	Difference between P_1 and P_2									
	0.05	0.10	0.15	0.20	0.25	0.30	0.35	0.40	0.45	0.50
0.05	473	159	88	59	43	33	26	22	18	16
0.10	724	219	112	72	51	37	29	24	20	17
0.15	944	270	133	82	57	41	32	26	21	18
0.20	1133	313	151	91	62	44	34	27	22	18
0.25	1289	348	165	98	66	47	35	28	22	18
0.30	1415	376	175	103	68	48	36	28	22	18
0.35	1509	395	182	106	69	48	36	28	22	18
0.40	1572	407	186	107	69	48	35	27	21	17
0.45	1603	411	186	106	68	47	34	26	20	16
0.50	1603	407	182	103	66	44	32	24	18	—
0.55	1572	395	175	98	62	41	29	22	—	—
0.60	1509	376	165	91	57	37	26	—	—	—
0.65	1415	348	151	82	51	33	—	—	—	—
0.70	1289	313	133	72	43	—	—	—	—	—
0.75	1133	270	112	59	—	—	—	—	—	—
0.80	944	219	88	—	—	—	—	—	—	—
0.85	724	159	—	—	—	—	—	—	—	—
0.90	473	—	—	—	—	—	—	—	—	—

Table 6.A1(c)   Sample size group for comparing two proportions (0.05–0.90 and 0.05–0.50) for a two-tailed hypothesis for $\alpha = 0.05$ and $\beta = 0.10$.

Least P	Difference between P_1 and P_2									
	0.05	0.10	0.15	0.20	0.25	0.30	0.35	0.40	0.45	0.50
0.05	620	207	113	75	54	41	33	27	23	19
0.10	958	286	146	92	65	48	37	30	25	21
0.15	1252	354	174	106	73	53	42	33	26	22
0.20	1504	412	197	118	80	57	44	34	27	23
0.25	1714	459	216	127	85	60	46	35	28	23
0.30	1883	496	230	134	88	62	47	36	28	23
0.35	2009	522	239	138	90	62	47	35	27	22
0.40	2093	538	244	139	90	62	46	34	26	21
0.45	2135	543	244	138	88	60	44	33	25	19
0.50	2135	538	239	134	85	57	42	30	23	—
0.55	2093	522	230	127	80	53	37	27	—	—
0.60	2009	496	216	118	73	48	33	—	—	—
0.65	1883	459	197	106	65	41	—	—	—	—
0.70	1714	412	174	92	54	—	—	—	—	—
0.75	1504	354	146	75	—	—	—	—	—	—
0.80	1252	286	113	—	—	—	—	—	—	—
0.85	958	207	—	—	—	—	—	—	—	—
0.90	620	—	—	—	—	—	—	—	—	—

Table 6.A1(d)   Sample size group for comparing two proportions (0.05–0.90 and 0.05–0.50) for a two-tailed hypothesis for $\alpha = 0.10$ and $\beta = 0.20$.

Least P	Difference between P_1 and P_2									
	0.01	0.02	0.03	0.04	0.05	0.06	0.07	0.08	0.09	0.10
0.01	2 019	700	396	271	204	162	134	114	98	87
0.02	3 205	994	526	343	249	193	157	131	113	97
0.03	4 367	1 283	653	414	294	224	179	148	126	109
0.04	5 505	1 564	777	482	337	254	201	165	139	119
0.05	6 616	1 838	898	549	380	283	222	181	151	129
0.06	7 703	2 107	1 016	615	422	312	243	197	163	139
0.07	8 765	2 369	1 131	680	463	340	263	212	175	148
0.08	9 803	2 627	1 244	743	502	367	282	227	187	158
0.09	10 816	2 877	1 354	804	541	393	302	241	198	167
0.10	11 804	3 121	1 461	863	578	419	320	255	209	175

Table 6.A1(e)   Sample size group for comparing two proportions (0.05–0.90 and 0.05–0.50) for a two-tailed hypothesis for $\alpha = 0.05$ and $\beta = 0.20$.

Least P	Difference between P_1 and P_2									
	0.01	0.02	0.03	0.04	0.05	0.06	0.07	0.08	0.09	0.10
0.01	2 512	864	487	332	249	197	163	138	120	106
0.02	4 018	1 237	651	423	306	238	192	161	137	120
0.03	5 493	1 602	813	512	363	276	220	182	154	133
0.04	6 935	1 959	969	600	419	314	248	203	170	146
0.05	8 347	2 308	1 123	686	473	351	275	223	186	159
0.06	9 726	2 650	1 272	769	526	388	301	243	202	171
0.07	11 076	2 983	1 419	850	577	423	327	263	217	183
0.08	12 393	3 308	1 562	930	627	457	352	282	232	195
0.09	13 679	3 626	1 702	1 007	676	491	377	300	246	207
0.10	14 933	3 936	1 838	1 083	724	523	401	318	260	218

Table 6.A1(f)   Sample size group for comparing two proportions (0.01–0.10 and 0.01–0.10) for a two-tailed hypothesis for $\alpha = 0.05$ and $\beta = 0.10$.

Least P	Difference between P_1 and P_2									
	0.01	0.02	0.03	0.04	0.05	0.06	0.07	0.08	0.09	0.10
0.01	3 300	1 125	631	428	320	254	209	178	154	135
0.02	5 320	1 625	852	550	397	307	248	207	177	154
0.03	7 296	2 114	1 067	671	474	359	286	236	199	172
0.04	9 230	2 593	1 277	788	548	410	323	264	221	189
0.05	11 123	3 061	1 482	902	620	460	360	291	242	206
0.06	12 973	3 518	1 684	1 014	691	508	395	318	263	223
0.07	14 780	3 965	1 880	1 123	760	555	429	343	283	239
0.08	16 546	4 401	2 072	1 229	827	602	463	369	303	255
0.09	18 270	4 827	2 259	1 333	893	647	495	393	322	270
0.10	19 952	5 242	2 441	1 434	957	690	527	417	341	285

Appendix 6.2: Tables for estimating the sample sizes when comparing the means from two groups

The standardized effect size (E/SD) is calculated by dividing the expected effect size (E) by the standard deviation (SD) of the effect variable.

To estimate the sample size use the table for the desired α (*P* value threshold) and select the appropriate standardized effect size row from the left-hand column; choose the appropriate column for the required β values and obtain the sample size at the intersection. If a one-tailed hypothesis is being tested, the α value can be halved (i.e. the $\alpha = 0.10$ for a two-tailed test given in the table provide the group sizes for $\alpha = 0.05$ for a one-tailed test).

Table 6.A2(b)   Sample size per group for comparing two means for a two-tailed hypothesis for $\alpha = 0.05$.

E/SD	$\beta = 0.05$	$\beta = 0.10$	$\beta = 0.20$
0.10	2600	2103	1571
0.15	1157	935	699
0.20	651	527	394
0.25	417	338	253
0.30	290	235	176
0.40	164	133	100
0.50	105	86	64
0.60	74	60	45
0.70	55	44	34
0.80	42	34	26
0.90	34	27	21
1.00	27	23	17

Table 6.A2(a)   Sample size per group for comparing two means for a two-tailed hypothesis for $\alpha = 0.01$.

E/SD	$\beta = 0.05$	$\beta = 0.10$	$\beta = 0.20$
0.10	3565	2978	2338
0.15	1586	1325	1040
0.20	893	746	586
0.25	572	478	376
0.30	398	333	262
0.40	225	188	148
0.50	145	121	96
0.60	101	85	67
0.70	75	63	50
0.80	58	49	39
0.90	46	39	21
1.00	38	32	26

Table 6.A2(c)   Sample size per group for comparing two means for a two-tailed hypothesis for $\alpha = 0.10$.

E/SD	$\beta = 0.05$	$\beta = 0.10$	$\beta = 0.20$
0.10	2166	1714	1238
0.15	963	762	551
0.20	542	429	310
0.25	347	275	199
0.30	242	191	139
0.40	136	108	78
0.50	88	70	51
0.60	61	49	36
0.70	45	36	26
0.80	35	28	21
0.90	28	22	16
1.00	23	18	14

Appendix 6.3: Tables for estimating the sample size to obtain the value of a proportion

Select the table with the desired confidence level (90%, 95% or 99%). From the left-hand column choose the row with the expected proportion. Select the column with the desired maximum width of the confidence interval and obtain the sample size estimate from the intersection of the row and column.

Table 6.A3(b)   Table for estimating the sample size to obtain the value of a proportion with a 95% confidence level.

Expected proportion	Total width of confidence interval						
	0.10	0.15	0.20	0.25	0.30	0.35	0.40
0.10	138	61	—	—	—	—	—
0.15	196	87	49	31	—	—	—
0.20	246	109	61	39	27	20	—
0.25	288	128	72	46	32	24	18
0.30	323	143	81	52	36	26	20
0.40	369	164	92	59	41	30	23
0.50	384	171	96	61	43	31	24

Table 6.A3(a)   Table for estimating the sample size to obtain the value of a proportion with a 90% confidence level.

Expected proportion	Total width of confidence interval						
	0.10	0.15	0.20	0.25	0.30	0.35	0.40
0.10	98	44	—	—	—	—	—
0.15	139	62	35	22	—	—	—
0.20	174	77	44	28	19	14	—
0.25	204	91	51	33	23	17	13
0.30	229	102	57	37	25	19	14
0.40	261	116	65	42	29	21	16
0.50	272	121	68	44	30	22	17

Table 6.A3(c)   Table for estimating the sample size to obtain the value of a proportion with a 99% confidence level.

Expected proportion	Total width of confidence interval						
	0.10	0.15	0.20	0.25	0.30	0.35	0.40
0.10	239	106	—	—	—	—	—
0.15	339	151	85	54	—	—	—
0.20	426	189	107	68	47	35	—
0.25	499	222	125	80	55	41	31
0.30	559	249	140	89	62	46	35
0.40	639	284	160	102	71	52	40
0.50	666	296	166	107	74	54	42

Appendix 6.4: Table for estimating a sample size to obtain a value for a continuous variable with a particular confidence width

The standardized width of the confidence interval expressed as a proportion of standard deviation (W/σ) should be calculated and used to select the appropriate row from the values given in the left-hand column. One of three levels of confidence can be selected (90%, 95% or 99%) to obtain the sample size required.

Table 6.A4

Standardized width	Confidence probability		
	90%	95%	99%
0.10	1083	1537	2665
0.15	482	683	1180
0.20	271	385	664
0.25	174	246	425
0.30	121	171	295
0.35	89	126	217
0.40	68	97	166
0.50	44	62	107
0.60	31	43	74
0.70	23	32	55
0.80	17	25	42
0.90	14	19	33
1.00	11	16	27

Appendix 6.5: Tables for estimating sample sizes for studies determining if correlation coefficients differ from zero

Choose the table that has the appropriate α value required. Select the lowest expected correlation coefficient that the study should be able to discriminate from no correlation (a correlation coefficient of zero) from the left-hand column and then obtain the sample size from the column headed by the chosen β value.

Table 6.A5(a) Table for estimating sample sizes for studies determining if correlation coefficients differ from zero for $\alpha = 0.1$.

Expected correlation coefficient	β value		
	0.05	0.10	0.20
0.05	7118	5947	4663
0.10	1773	1481	1162
0.15	783	655	514
0.20	436	365	287
0.25	276	231	182
0.30	189	158	125
0.35	136	114	90
0.40	102	86	68
0.45	79	66	53
0.50	62	52	42
0.60	40	34	27
0.70	27	23	19
0.80	18	15	13

Table 6.A5(b) Table for estimating sample sizes for studies determining if correlation coefficients differ from zero for $\alpha = 0.05$.

Expected correlation coefficient	β value		
	0.05	0.10	0.20
0.05	5193	4200	3134
0.10	1294	1047	782
0.15	572	463	346
0.20	319	259	194
0.25	202	164	123
0.30	139	113	85
0.35	100	82	62
0.40	75	62	47
0.45	58	48	36
0.50	46	38	29
0.60	30	25	19
0.70	20	17	13
0.80	14	12	9

Table 6.A5(c) Table for estimating sample sizes for studies determining if correlation coefficients differ from zero for $\alpha = 0.01$.

Expected correlation coefficient	β value		
	0.05	0.10	0.20
0.05	4325	3424	2469
0.10	1078	854	616
0.15	477	378	273
0.20	266	211	153
0.25	169	134	98
0.30	116	92	67
0.35	84	67	49
0.40	63	51	37
0.45	49	39	29
0.50	39	31	23
0.60	26	21	16
0.70	17	14	11
0.80	12	10	8

COHORT STUDIES

Objectives

After reading this chapter readers should:

- be able to recognize when a cohort study would be appropriate
- understand the advantages and disadvantages of cohort studies
- understand variations of cohort study designs
- be able to design and implement a cohort study.

7.1   Introduction

Like experimental studies, observational studies are explanatory in nature, with a comparison between two groups. However, unlike experimental studies the allocation of the study animals to the groups being compared is not under the control of the researcher, although matching of the individuals selected for the study is. The power of the study is therefore diminished.

Observational studies allow investigations to be performed that may be practically impossible to perform experimentally. For example, studies regarding body condition scores and fertility in cattle would be very expensive to study by experiment, yet relatively inexpensive to study by observational designs. This type of study is often used to investigate risk factors in disease, for example the development of urolithiasis and different types of cat food. There are three broad groups of observational studies: cohort, cross-sectional and case-control. Cohort studies are sometimes used to generate a life table that can be used for prognosis.

7.2   Cohort studies

A cohort study is a study in which animals exposed to a putative causal factor are followed over time and compared with another group who are not exposed to that factor with regard to a specified health outcome. Prognosis, treatment and causation can be studied using cohort studies.

The two groups are equally monitored for specific outcomes. Alternatively, two or more different treatments may be compared. Both groups contain animals which have the disease under investigation, and each group receives one of the treatments. This type of study allows comparison of risk and intervention. For example, dogs with an amputated hind leg could be monitored for the development of osteoarthritis in the remaining hind leg over a 24-month period. These animals would be compared to a group of healthy dogs. Matching the affected group to the control group is important to reduce any variables other than the factor of interest between the groups.

Cohort studies can be prospective or retrospective. Prospective studies follow two groups of subjects within the sample from the population. One group has a potential risk factor present and the other group does not. Both groups are monitored over time for the development of a disease of interest or at a specific follow-up time for the presence of the disease (Fig. 7.1). Retrospective studies identify two groups within the sample of subjects from the population: one group with and one without the risk factor of interest. The records are examined for the occurrence of disease within the individuals in the groups (Fig. 7.2).

7.2.1   Advantages

- Cohort studies are generally preferred to case-control studies as they are statistically more reliable. They are also cheaper than randomized controlled trials.
- Compared to case-control studies, cohort studies can establish the timing and sequence of events.
- In prospective studies data collection can be standardized in comparison to the use of historical records.
- Cohort studies are powerful at demonstrating causality.
- Cohort studies allow several diseases to be studied simultaneously.

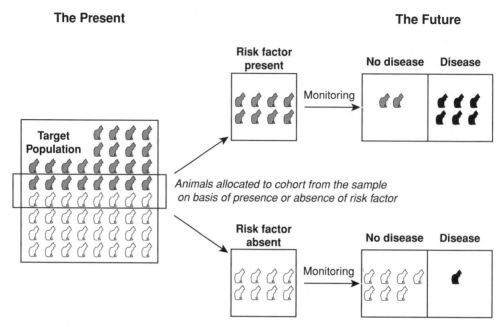

Figure 7.1 Schematic representation of a prospective cohort study.

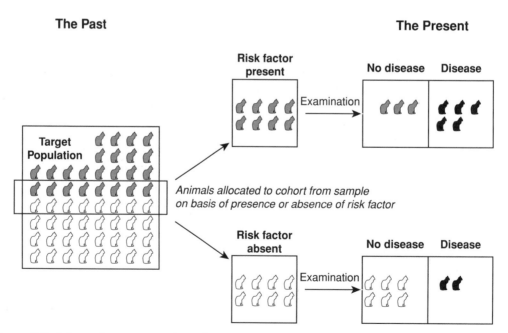

Figure 7.2 Schematic representation of a retrospective cohort study.

7.2.2 *Disadvantages*

- Blinding is difficult and identifying a matched control group to minimize other variables can be difficult.
- Cohort studies are not as reliable as randomized controlled studies as the two groups may differ in ways other than the variable under study.
- Cohort studies can take a long time to complete and there may be a loss of participants (dropout bias).
- Cohort studies are not useful for rare diseases and those that require a long period of exposure to the predisposing factor of interest. It is very expensive and time-consuming to monitor a large cohort of subjects over a long period.
- Exposure to the factor of interest may change over time, which can make the analysis more complicated and reduce the power of the experiment.
- Behaviour may be altered by being part of the study and confound the results.

7.2.3 *Measures of risks in cohort studies*

The results are usually expressed in terms of the strength of the association between the risk factor and outcome, and the statistical significance of this association. Relative risk is the ratio of incidence in exposed individuals to the incidence in non-exposed individuals. If there is no difference in risk regarding the outcome then the ratio is equal to 1. Relative risk is an index of the strength of association between exposure and disease. Attributable risk (absolute risk) is the difference between the disease incidences of the exposed and unexposed groups and is the incidence of disease attributable to exposure to the risk factor.

Population attributable risk is a measure of how much a risk factor contributes to disease incidence at the population level. It is the product of the attributable risk and the prevalence of the risk factor in the population.

Population attributable fraction is the proportion of the disease in the population that is accounted for by virtue of the presence of the risk factor. It is simply the population attributable risk divided by the total incidence of the disease in the population.

7.3 Prospective cohort studies

A prospective study is one that is conducted forwards in time with the subjects classified into groups depending on whether or not they are exposed to a risk factor. In a prospective cohort study the investigator selects or defines a sample of subjects. A characteristic (risk factor) is measured that may have an association or predictive value for a given outcome (disease). The subjects are followed over time and periodic measurements of the outcome of interest are made. Ideally all the animals entering the study should be free of the disease being studied. During the follow-up the incidence is recorded.

The exposed and non-exposed subjects are compared with regard to the rates of development of an outcome of interest. This comparison between exposed and non-exposed groups enables the strength of the relationship between a risk factor and an outcome to be determined. In addition, evidence regarding the dose-effect relationship between the risk and outcome may be deduced. The temporal relationship between the risk factor and the outcome may be available if multiple follow-up measurements have been performed throughout the follow-up period. Prognostic information may be produced if the outcome is fatal and a life table is produced. Useful estimates of the incidence of disease within the population can be generated. The results may demonstrate harm or benefit.

7.3.1 *Strengths*

Prospective cohort study design is a powerful strategy for defining the incidence and investigating the potential predisposing and causative factors. Important variables can be accurately measured without reliance on records or memory. The presence of the factors or absence of the factors is established before the onset of disease, thus increasing the inference of a causal association. Recall bias is absent because events are recorded as they occur. In most cases it is clear that the exposure came before the disease (the exception being diseases with long incubation periods that are difficult to detect in the preclinical phase).

7.3.2   Weaknesses

Prospective cohort study design is not well suited to conditions that are rare. The number of subjects that need to be followed to obtain a prerequisite number of outcomes is large and the study becomes expensive and inefficient. Diseases with long incubation periods or which require prolonged exposure to a risk factor before being detected require expensive, long follow-up periods. The long follow-up period also results in increased dropout rates.

7.4   Retrospective cohort studies

The design of the retrospective cohort study is essentially the same as the prospective study but differs in that the follow-up and outcomes happened in the past. This study can only be performed if this historical information is available.

7.4.1   Strengths

The variable measurements cannot be biased by prior knowledge of the outcome. They are less costly than prospective studies as the follow-up period has already taken place and if records are being used the measurements of outcomes have already been performed. This type of study is an efficient approach to research when the disease under study has a prolonged course and there may be many potential hypotheses regarding the causation. Retrospective cohort studies are useful when the disease is rare and/or the disease has a prolonged latency period.

7.4.2   Weaknesses

The investigator has limited control over the sampling of the population and the factors that can be studied. The type and quality of the measurements cannot be predetermined. Records of subjects and items of information that are important to answering the research may not be available. The ability and motivation of owners to recall past exposure to a risk factor is sometimes related to whether their animal did or did not have the outcome. This results in recall bias. Ascertaining the time sequence of exposure and outcome can be difficult with retrospective studies, which weakens the evidence for causality.

7.5   Combined prospective and retrospective survival cohort studies across time and place

A survival cohort is a group of individuals who are often at different stages in their disease rather than at the onset at the start of the study.

Although less than ideal, circumstances may arise when useful information can be derived from using data from both types of study on the same topic. In medicine it may become unethical to withhold a treatment although quantification of the benefit is lacking. An example using a survival cohort to examine the effect on taurine supplementation in cats diagnosed with dilated cardiomyopathy is described by Smith (2006). A prospective study recording the survival of cats diagnosed with this condition and then supplemented with taurine is compared to the survival of cats with this condition from a retrospective study on cats that historically received no supplementation. The comparison indicates the benefit derived from the supplementation in terms of increased survival times.

7.6   Nested case-control and case cohort studies

7.6.1   Nested case-control studies

The nested case-control study (see Figure 7.3) has a case-control study embedded within either

**Measurements in the present
from samples from the past**

The Present

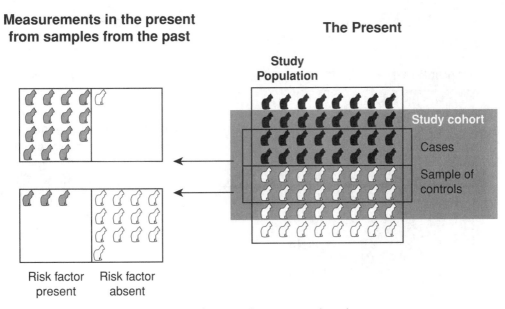

Study
Population

Study cohort

Cases

Sample of
controls

Risk factor   Risk factor
present   absent

Figure 7.3 Schematic representation of a nested case-control study.

a prospective or retrospective cohort study. It is the design of choice for variables that are expensive to measure and that can be measured at the end of the study from appropriately stored samples taken before the onset of the outcome of interest.

In case-control studies subjects confirmed with the disease (cases) are compared with non-diseased subjects (control subjects) regarding past exposure to a putative risk factor (variable). The design of a case-control study may or may not involve a matching procedure. In matched case-control studies each unexposed control subject is matched in some way to a case subject. The matching criteria involve potential confounding factors.

A cohort of subjects from a population is followed (prospectively or retrospectively). The investigator identifies all the members of the cohort who have developed the outcome (disease) of interest. This group is known as the cases. An appropriate sample of the cohort subjects who did not develop the outcome is selected as the case-control group.

The investigator then measures the appropriate variables for the cases and case-control groups using the stored material (e.g. serum, semen, biopsies, radiographs). The values of the variables for the two groups can then be compared.

7.6.2 Nested case-cohort

In this design a random sample of all the members of the cohort is taken and their baseline stored samples are analysed. A proportion will have the outcome of interest (cases) and the complement will not (controls). One advantage of this design is that one sample can provide the controls for several case-control studies, each using a different outcome. Because the sample is randomly selected, the prevalence of the risk factor in the population can be estimated from the results of the variable measurements from the stored samples.

This is a cost-effective design when the measurement of variables is expensive.

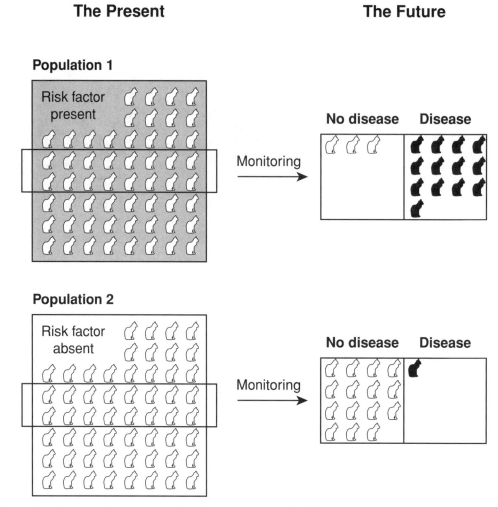

Figure 7.4 Schematic representation of a prospective double cohort study.

7.7   Multiple-cohort studies

The investigator selects samples from populations with different levels of the variable (as illustrated in Figure 7.4). This can be prospective or retrospective. The outcomes in the two samples are compared.

7.7.1   Strengths

This is a useful design for studying exposures to rare risk factors.

7.7.2   Weaknesses

Because the cohorts are from different populations there may be other differences between the populations that can confound the results.

7.8   Planning a cohort study

Cohort studies follow patients through time to determine what becomes of them. This study design is often used to demonstrate associations between suspected causes and disease.

The animals which form the cohort should be appropriate to the research question and available for the follow-up. They should be representative of the population. The number selected should be based on the power required.

The outcomes should be assessed using appropriate case definitions and the investigator should be blinded to the values of the variable under investigation. Ideally the investigator should be able to follow the entire cohort. This should be carefully considered when participants are being selected.

7.8.1 Checklist for cohort study designs

Are the exposure criteria described?

The criteria by which subjects are assessed as being exposed or non-exposed to a risk factor need to be clearly defined. These criteria should be set before the selection process.

If it is relevant, the different grades of exposure to the risk factor should be recorded so that the dose-effect relationships between the risk factor and the outcome may be examined.

Will exposure be monitored and recorded throughout the follow-up period?

Subjects assessed as being unexposed at the start of the study may become exposed to the putative risk factor during the study. Similarly, exposed subjects confirmed as being exposed to the risk factor at the start of the study may cease to be exposed in a later part of the study. Measures to identify and record these changes in exposure should be part of the study protocol and appear in the study report. If they are ignored the conclusion may be invalid.

How will the subjects be selected?

The subjects should be representative of the target population. The unexposed group should be similar in all other respects to the exposed group.

Is the outcome variable objective and easy to measure?

Outcomes should be measured in the same way in both the exposed and unexposed groups, and the investigator should be blinded to their membership of these categories.

Will the exposed and non-exposed groups be subject to the same range of variables?

Factors that may have an impact on the outcome measure other than the variable under investigation should be measured and recorded for the two groups so that these differences can be taken into account in the analysis.

Will the exposed and unexposed groups be similar?

The compared groups must be generally similar with regard to characteristics that may have an influence on the outcome, for example breed, sex, and age. In small samples the power of the study may be increased by matching but this process must be taken into account when performing the statistical appraisal.

Is the follow-up period adequate?

The follow-up period should be sufficiently long to enable a predetermined difference in outcome to be identified. This is not always easy to predict unless previous knowledge or pilot trials enable estimates to be derived. The time boundaries may have to be set by a reasonable time frame that has clinical significance.

How will subjects that drop out be handled?

Dropouts should be minimized by careful selection of participants. However, detailed descriptions of subjects that drop out should be kept so that any systematic differences between these and the subjects completing the trial can be examined for bias.

How is the sample size to be determined?

The size of the cohort study will be determined by the prevalence of the disorder and the magnitude of the risk posed by exposure to the putative risk factor. A larger cohort is required for rare diseases or when the risk associated with the putative risk factor is low.

Here are some questions a reviewer may ask about your study. It is useful to consider whether your experimental design would stand up to this scrutiny.

1. Did the study address a clearly focused issue?
   - What is the population being studied?
   - What risk factors are being studied?
   - What outcomes are being considered?
   - Is the study trying to detect harmful or beneficial effects?
2. Is a cohort study a good way of answering the question?
3. Was the exposure/outcome accurately measured to minimize bias?
4. Who exactly has been recruited to the study? (Was there selection bias?)
   - Was the cohort representative of the defined population?
   - Was there anything special about the cohort members?
5. How was the sample size determined? Was a power calculation performed?
6. Was the follow-up of all subjects complete? Those lost to follow-up can bias a study if they do better or worse than those that remain and more are lost from one group than another.
7. Were all subjects examined with equal intensity?
8. Were the data on outcomes collected identically in both groups? Were the observers doing the measurements blinded?
9. Have the authors identified all the important confounding factors? (Were the compared groups similar?)
10. Were other factors affecting the outcome other than the one of interest (e.g. age, sex,

breed) either equally distributed in the outcome groups or controlled by the method of analysis? If not, could the difference in these other factors account for the outcome observed?
11. Was the follow-up of subjects long enough regarding the known facts about the natural history of the disease? For example, has the treatment or exposure been long enough to demonstrate a measurable effect?
12. Are the comparisons unbiased? To attribute outcome to the factor of interest other determinants of the outcome must occur equally in the groups compared.
13. Does the relationship identified or studied make biological and chronological sense?
14. How strong is the association and how precise is the estimate?
15. Has the target population been described in detail?

7.8.2   Reporting the results of a cohort study

The results of a cohort study are conventionally reported in the form of a relative risk or risk ratio (see Figure 7.5). Relative risk is the ratio of the experimental event rate to the control event rate and is used to quantify the difference in risk between the two groups.

$$RR = \frac{EER}{CER}$$

A RR below 1 shows there is less chance of the event happening in the experimental group, and a RR above 1 shows there is a greater chance. Again there is no reference to the baseline risk, and therefore the absolute benefit to be gained.

7.8.3   Examples

Example 1: Prospective cohort study

Risk factors associated with diarrhoea in newborn calves (Bendali et al., 1999)

A prospective study was carried out on 94 randomly selected beef calf herds in the Midi-Pyrenees region in France in order to determine

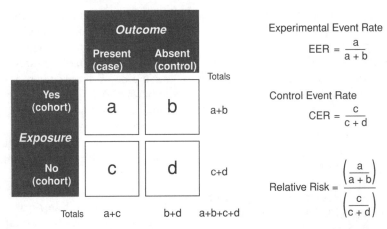

Figure 7.5 Contingency table illustrating the method for calculating relative risk.

neonatal gastroenteritis risk factors. A total of 3,080 newborn calves was enrolled from December 1995 to April 1996. By using a specific statistical analysis method that takes into account an 'intra-herd' correlation, our final model allows the identification of approximately 20 management risk factors associated with diarrhoea. We confirmed several factors identified previously (calving conditions) and estimated some new factors (month of birth). Several herd level factors were found to be significantly associated with the risk of diarrhoea. These factors included herd management conditions such as hygiene (cleaning, relative risk (RR) = 1.9), and also vitamin or salt supplements to animals and cow vaccination (RR = 2). It was found amongst the calf level factors, that calving conditions and dyspnea were associated with diarrhoea. Dam vaccination seemed to protect calves against illness. A relationship between diarrhoea and the month of birth was also observed. Our results confirmed that calf diarrhoea is a multifactor pathology and prevention should be considered globally within the farm.

Example 2: A retrospective study

Retrospective study of the risk factors and prevalence of colic in horses after orthopaedic surgery (Senior et al., 2004)

The records of 496 orthopaedic operations on 428 horses were reviewed to estimate the prevalence of, and identify the risk factors for, the development of colic in horses after surgery. Colic was defined as any recognised sign of abdominal pain that could not be attributed to a concurrent disease. Fourteen of the horses developed colic; eight of them were undiagnosed, three were classified as impactions, one as tympanic colic of the colon, one as incarceration of the small intestine in the epiploic foramen, and one as left dorsal displacement of the colon in the nephrosplenic space. Morphine was associated with a four-fold increased risk of colic compared with the use of no opioid or butorphanol, and out-of-hours surgery was also associated with an increased risk.

7.9 Cohort studies and prognosis

Prognosis is a prediction of the course of disease following its onset. Studies of prognosis have much in common with studies on risk. A group of animals with a specified condition are assembled and followed forwards over time and the clinical outcomes measured.

Participating individual subjects who form the cohort in prognostic studies are observed from a starting point called zero time. Ideally this point should be at the same or clearly defined stage in the course of the disease in all subjects. If the observations begin at different stages in the course of the disease for different individuals then the relative time course of events such as recovery, recurrence and death will be more difficult to interpret and describe.

Rates that have been used to describe prognosis include the survival rate (the percentage of patients that survive a defined period of time from some point in the course of the disease), the case fatality rate (the percentage of patients with the disease who die of it), the response rate (the percentage of patients showing some improvement following an intervention), the remission rate (the percentage of patients in which the disease is no longer detectable) and the recurrence rate (the percentage of patients who experience a return of disease after a disease-free interval) (Fletcher et al., 1996). However, these summary rates usually do not provide the mean likelihood of an event that a patient with a condition will experience at a certain point in time. Survival curves or life table analysis are used to obtain these values.

7.10   Summary

1. In cohort studies, subjects are followed over time in order to describe the incidence or natural history of disease and to analyse variables (risk factors) for various outcomes. Measuring the predictor before the outcome occurs indicates the sequence of events and helps to control bias in that measurement.
2. Prospective cohort studies on rare conditions are likely to require large numbers of subjects followed for a long period of time. The use of a retrospective cohort design by analysing records or samples that have already been collected may be an option.
3. The nested case-control study may be another effective study design. Samples or data are collected and stored until the end of the study; measurements are taken from

the stored materials for all animals that have developed the outcome of interest, and for a sample of those that have not.
4. The multiple-cohort design compares the incidence of disease (or other outcome) in cohorts that differ in the level of a predictor variable and may be used to study the effects of rare exposures.
5. Bias in the assessment of outcomes is prevented by standardizing the measurements and blinding them to the values of predictor variables.
6. The clinical value of the results from a cohort study can be reduced by poor follow-up of subjects. This can be avoided by excluding animals who are not likely to be available for follow-up.

7.11   References

Bendali F, Sanaa M, Bichet H, Schelcher F (1999) Risk factors associated with diarrhoea in newborn calves. *Vet. Res.* **30**(5): 509–22.

Fletcher RH, Fletcher SW, Wagner EH (1996) *Clinical Epidemiology (The Essentials)*, 3rd edn, Williams and Wilkins, Baltimore, p 117.

Senior JM, Pinchbeck GL, Dugdale AH, Clegg PD (2004) Retrospective study of the risk factors and prevalence of colic in horses after orthopaedic surgery. *Vet. Rec.* Sep 11 **155**(11): 321–5.

Smith RD (2006) Design and evaluation of clinical trials. In: *Veterinary Clinical Epidemiology*, 3rd edn, CRC Press, London, pp 130–1.

7.12   Further reading

Ajetunmobi O (2002) Critical appraisal of prospective studies. In: *Making Sense of Critical Appraisal*, Arnold, London, pp 100–11.

Ajetunmobi O (2002) Critical appraisal of retrospective studies. In: *Making Sense of Critical Appraisal*, Arnold, London, pp 112–21.

Ajetunmobi O (2002) Handling survival time data. In: *Making Sense of Critical Appraisal*, Arnold, London, pp 146–53.

Dahoo IR, Waltner-Toews D (1985) Interpreting Clinical Research: Part I. General Considerations. *Compendium of Continuing Education* **7**(9); S474–S477.

Dahoo IR, Waltner-Toews D (1985) Interpreting Clinical Research: Part II. Descriptive and Experimental Studies. *Compendium of Continuing Education* **7**(9); S513–S519.

Dahoo IR, Waltner-Toews D (1985) Interpreting Clinical Research: Part 1. Observational Studies and Interpretation of Results. *Compendium of Continuing Education* **7**(9); S605–S613.

Fletcher RH, Fletcher SW, Wagner EH (1996) *Risk in Clinical Epidemiology (The Essentials)*, 3rd edn, Williams and Wilkins, Baltimore, pp 94–110.

Fletcher RH, Fletcher SW, Wagner EH (1996) *Prognosis in Clinical Epidemiology (The Essentials)*, 3rd edn, Williams and Wilkins, Baltimore, pp 111–35.

Hulley SB, Cummings SR, Warren SB, Grady DG, Newman TB (2007) Designing a Cohort Study. In: *Designing Clinical Research*, 3rd edn, Lippincott Williams and Wilkins, Philadelphia, pp 97–108.

Smith RD (2006) Risk assessment and prevention. In: *Veterinary Clinical Epidemiology*, 3rd edn, CRC Press, London, pp 91–109.

Smith RD (2006) Design and evaluation of clinical trials. In: *Veterinary Clinical Epidemiology*, 3rd edn, CRC Press, London, pp 127–37.

Thrusfield M (2005) Observational studies. In: *Veterinary Epidemiology*, 3rd edn, Blackwell Publishing, Oxford, pp 266–88.

Woodward M (2005) Cohort studies. In: *Epidemiology: Study and Data Analysis*, Chapman and Hall/CRC, London, pp 215–72.

7.13 MCQs

1 *Cohort studies are:*

(a) observational studies
(b) useful to study a putative risk factor and the development of a specified disease
(c) useful to compare one or more preventative treatments
(d) usually less expensive than clinical trials
(e) useful for all the above reasons.

2 *Prospective studies:*

(a) are conducted forwards in time
(b) are conducted backwards in time
(c) do not monitor outcomes
(d) usually use records
(e) collect non-specific data.

3 *Retrospective studies:*

(a) are conducted forwards in time
(b) are conducted backwards in time
(c) only include animals that have developed the disease of interest
(d) do not usually use records
(e) only include animals that have been exposed to the putative risk factor.

4 *Which of the following is a strength of prospective studies?*

(a) Important variables can be accurately measured without reliance on records or memory.
(b) They are useful to study rare conditions.
(c) They are useful to study conditions with a long incubation period.
(d) They are useful to study risk factors that are expensive to measure.
(e) All of the above.

5 *Which of the following is a weakness of prospective studies?*

(a) Measurement of variables relies on historical records or memory.
(b) They are not useful to study rare conditions.
(c) They cannot be used to estimate the incidence of a specified disease in the population.
(d) Measuring the exposure to the putative factor is difficult.
(e) It is impossible to determine the time sequence of exposure and outcome.

6 *Which of the following is a strength of retrospective studies?*

(a) They are useful to study rare conditions.
(b) The type and quality of the measurements cannot be predetermined.
(c) Measurement of variables rely on historical records or memory.
(d) Recall bias is not a problem.
(e) They are more expensive than prospective studies.

7 *Which of the following is a weakness of retrospective studies?*

(a) They are not useful to study rare conditions.
(b) The type and quality of the measurements cannot be predetermined.
(c) They are more expensive than prospective studies.
(d) The cost of the study is difficult to determine.
(e) Lost to follow-up subjects is a problem.

8 *Nested case-control studies are advantageous when:*

(a) measurement of the variable is expensive
(b) measurement of the variable is inexpensive
(c) outcomes are not easily identified
(d) more power is needed in the study
(e) cases cannot be identified.

9 *Nested case-cohort studies are useful for:*

(a) investigating more than one variable and outcome
(b) cost reduction
(c) measuring the prevalence of the risk factor
(d) when studying rare events
(e) all of the above.

10 *Multiple cohort studies are useful for:*

(a) common diseases
(b) common risk factors
(c) multiple risk factors
(d) rare risk factors
(e) studies where time is limited.

7.14 MCQ answers

1. (e); 2. (a); 3. (b); 4. (a); 5. (b); 6. (a); 7. (b); 8. (a); 9. (d); 10. (d)

8

CROSS-SECTIONAL AND CASE-CONTROL STUDIES

Objectives

After reading this chapter readers should:

- understand the advantages and disadvantages of cross-sectional and case-control studies
- be able to recognize when these study designs are appropriate
- be able to plan and implement cross-sectional and case-control studies.

8.1   Introduction

Chapter 7 on cohort studies described how measurements follow the time sequence of cause and effect. This chapter describes two types of observational study that do not follow this time sequence. In a cross-sectional study all the measurements are made 'simultaneously' in the present. In case-control studies the investigator works backwards in time. The predictor variables in the case and control groups are compared to investigate the association with the specified outcome.

Both types of study identifies a group with a specified disease and a group without a specified disease from a sample taken from a target population. The sensitivity and specificity of a diagnostic test can be measured using these groups. The evaluation of diagnostic tests is described in Chapter 10.

8.2   Cross-sectional studies

The structure of a cross-sectional study is similar to a cohort study except that all the measurements are made together without a follow-up period. Cohort studies can provide the incidence of disease whereas cross-sectional studies can only generate the prevalence of disease. Prevalence is a measure of the proportion of the population who have a specified disease at a point in time; incidence is the proportion of animals which get the disease over a period of time. Prevalence information is useful in assessing the importance of the disease and the likelihood of

patients having the disease. However, because incidence cannot be obtained this limits the information the cross-sectional study design can produce on prognosis, natural history and disease causation. A factor which is found to be associated with the prevalence of disease may not be a cause of the disease but may be simply be associated with the disease. For example, a thin ewe is associated with but not the cause of scrapie in sheep.

The data can be used to determine a relationship between exposure to a factor and presence of disease. A representative sample of the target population is selected. Within the sample two groups are identified, into those animals with a specified disease and those without. Identical sets of parameters (risk factor exposures) are then recorded for the two groups (Fig. 8.1). The strength of the relationship between the disease and the parameter can then be expressed as an odds ratio. This is the only type of study that can yield true prevalence rates. Cross-sectional studies are also appropriate for describing the distribution patterns of variables in a target population.

Serial cross-sectional surveys of a target population can be used to investigate changing patterns over time. This is not a cohort design as it does not follow a single group over time. This design avoids any bias caused by the impact that the measurements may have on the subjects.

8.2.1   Advantages

- Cross-sectional studies are relatively inexpensive and quick to perform.
- They present very few ethical problems.
- If a random sample is taken from the target population the disease/risk prevalence and the proportions of exposed and unexposed animals can be determined.
- More than one risk factor can be investigated and networks of causal links can be explored.

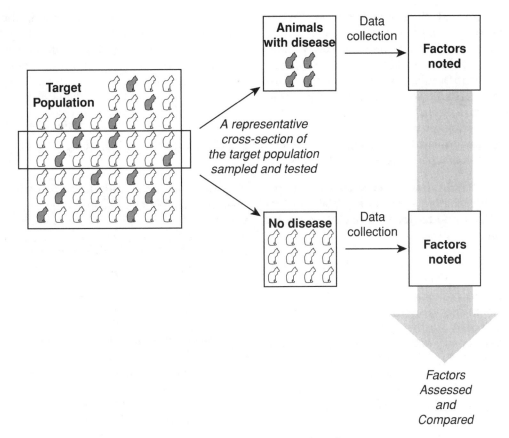

Figure 8.1 A schematic representation of a cross-sectional study.

8.2.2 Disadvantages

- Cross-sectional studies generate hypotheses, rather than test hypotheses.
- A cross-sectional study is an inappropriate design to study a rare disease, as the number of subjects required would be too great.
- The temporal relationship between risk and disease cannot be determined so the evidence for the causal link between the putative risk factor and outcome is usually weak or circumstantial.

8.2.3 Examples

The abstracts of two published papers using cross-sectional study designs are given below.

Epidemiological study of decubital ulcers in sows (Davies et al., 1996)

Objective: To determine prevalence and risk factors for decubital ulcers of the shoulder in sows. *Design*: Descriptive cross-sectional study. *Sample population*: All females of breeding age in a large confinement swine facility. *Procedure*: 1916 females were examined for lesions of the skin over the tuber of the spine of the scapula and for body condition scoring. Observational data were combined with sow data (parity, date of farrowing, litter size) contained in computerized records. *Results*: Decubital ulcers were observed in 8.3% of females, predominantly lactating sows. Ulcer prevalence was strongly associated with time after farrowing. Lesions apparently healed rapidly after weaning. Ulcer prevalence was associated with low body condition scores, but was not associated with parity. *Implications*: Decubital ulcers are a multifactorial condition. Housing on concrete floors per se did not result in ulcers. Prolonged recumbency during parturition, reduced activity in early lactation, periparturient illness, thin body condition, moist skin and floor type are potential risk factors.

Risk factors for porcine post-weaning multisystemic wasting syndrome (PMWS) in 149 French farrow-to-finish herds (Rose et al., 2003)

A cross-sectional study involving 149 farms was carried out in France in 2000 and 2001 to assess the risk factors for post-weaning multisystemic wasting syndrome (PMWS). The farms were divided into three groups according to their current or past PMWS status: cases (current and typical PMWS), controls#1 (PMWS-free farms), and controls#2 (farms which have recovered from PMWS). Two different comparisons were tested: cases versus controls#1, and cases versus controls#2. In the first comparison, the odds of PMWS were increased when fattening pigs tested positive for parvovirus (PPv) and porcine reproductive and respiratory syndrome (PRRS) virus (OR = 4.4 and 6.5, respectively), when separate vaccines for parvovirus and Erysipelas for the gilts versus associated vaccines were used (OR = 2.5) and when on-farm semen collection was used versus all the semen purchased from an insemination centre (OR = 4.6). Large pens in weaning facilities increased the odds of PMWS (OR = 4.1), whereas long empty periods in weaning and farrowing facilities versus shorter (OR = 0.2) regular treatment against external parasites (OR = 0.1) and housing the sows in collective pens during pregnancy versus individual pens (OR = 0.3) all decreased the odds of PMWS. The same kinds of risk factors were found with the second comparison with, in addition, a common pit for several adjacent fattening rooms versus separate pits (OR = 6.7) and a high level of cross-

fostering (OR = 5.1). On the other hand, when farms had a self-replacement scheme for the gilts (OR = 0.1), and when vaccination of the sows against *E. coli* was in place (OR = 0.2), the odds of PMWS were decreased.

8.2.4   Cross-sectional study design checklist

Is the study appropriate for the scientific question?

Cross-sectional surveys are descriptive studies in which a sample population's status is determined for the absence of exposure and disease at the same time. They are hypothesis generating rather than hypothesis testing. It can also be used to establish the true prevalence of a disease.

1. Is the target population be clearly defined?
2. Will the sample be representative of the population?
3. Is the sampling method valid (random)?
4. Could the result be time dependent (would a different result have been obtained at a different time of day/month/season?)
5. If a questionnaire is used could bias be introduced by the type of question or the literacy of the respondents? Could the responders as opposed to the non-responders bias the survey in any way?

8.3   Case-control studies

Cohort and cross-sectional studies to investigate the cause of disease in all but the most common diseases would have to be large and as a consequence they would be expensive. Case-control studies are an easier and less expensive alternative, which produce a high yield of information from relatively few subjects. They are an appropriate design for rare diseases or diseases with long latency periods between exposure to a risk factor and the development of disease. This design may be the only feasible option for some diseases; multiple putative variables can be explored and it is a useful design for generating hypotheses. Case-control studies can

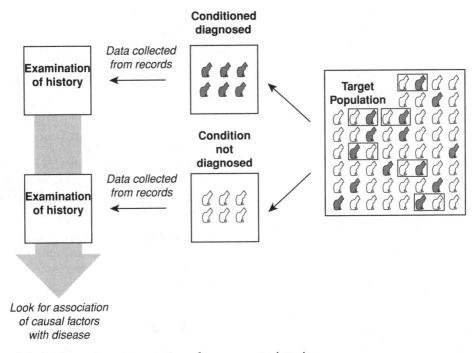

Figure 8.2 A schematic representation of a case-control study.

provide descriptive information on the characteristics of the cases and an estimate of the association between each putative variable and the presence or absence of disease. These estimates are in the form of odds ratios, which approximate to the relative risk if the prevalence of the disease is not too high. However, they also have their limitations. They cannot provide estimates of the incidence or prevalence of disease and they can only investigate one outcome. Cohort studies and cross-sectional studies can investigate more than one outcome variable. Case-control studies have an increased chance of bias, particularly from the separate sampling of the cases and controls and the retrospective measurement of putative risk variables.

Animals in a target population that have developed a disease condition are identified and their exposure to suspected causal or risk factors is compared with that of a control group who do not have the disease (Fig. 8.2). A case-control study is always retrospective as the information regarding exposure is historical. Risk factors may be investigated using this type of study by using a questionnaire. For example, the diets of dogs with osteochondritis dissecans (OCD) could be compared to dogs that do not have OCD, and their dietary and exercise histories recorded for a possible link. However, just because there is a statistical relationship between a risk factor and a condition, it does not necessarily mean that there is a causal relationship. Case-control studies can also be used to provide evidence of whether an intervention has been effective or not. The results are expressed as odds ratios. Absolute risk cannot be determined.

8.3.1 Design of a case-control study

1. The target population is identified.
2. Sample size is defined by a power calculation.

3. Cases of the disease (or clinical event) to be investigated are identified in the target population using clearly defined case definitions.
4. Controls are recruited from the target population and are matched for important confounding variables.
5. Assess the cases and controls for exposure to the risk factor being investigated. Blinding is advisable if possible.
6. Analyse the results (odds/relative risk).

8.3.2   Controlling sampling bias

Ideally the sample of cases would be a random sample of animals which has the disease in the target population. It is more likely the cases will consist of subjects diagnosed with the disease and who are readily available for the study. The sample may not be representative with respect to the putative risk factor and may introduce a bias in the cases recruited. Various strategies can be used to recruit appropriate controls. An important component of the experimental design is matching controls to cases. Controls should be chosen to be as similar as possible to the cases. Factors such as age, sex, breed, weight and diet, among other variables, may need to be matched if they have a perceived or actual impact on the value of the outcome measure. One of the problems of overmatching is finding enough controls and a balance may need to be struck. An important technique for increasing the power of the study is to enrol more than one control for every case. The use of two controls per case usually gives the greatest statistical advantage. Alternatively, if bias in the control groups is a concern then more than one control group can be selected from different settings.

8.3.3   Controlling measurement bias

Differential recall by owners with pets that have a condition and owners with pets that do not have a condition will result in bias. Accurate and systematic records can avoid bias. A further measurement bias may be introduced by the unblinded record analyst who is aware of the identification of controls and cases. It may be possible to blind the analyst to which group the records belong to and to which risk putative factor is being investigated.

Case-control studies are relatively quick, inexpensive and easy to perform. They are appropriate for studying rare diseases or outcomes. They do require complete and accurate standardized records. They are useful as a preliminary investigation of a suspected risk factor for a common condition or an adverse event related to an intervention.

They are useful to formulate hypotheses that can be tested using study designs higher up on the hierarchy, such as cohort or randomized controlled trials.

8.3.4   Advantages

- The main advantages are that these studies are quick to perform and do not require special methods to conduct.
- They are generally inexpensive and may be the only way in which rare conditions or those with a long incubation period can be realistically studied.
- They can be used to evaluate interventions as well as associations.
- Many risk factors can be studied simultaneously.
- They usually require smaller sample sizes than cohort studies.

8.3.5   Disadvantages

- Case-control studies are less reliable than either randomized controlled trials or cohort studies as it is difficult to match the control group and eliminate confounding variables.
- It is not possible to calculate true incidence/prevalence and relative risk.
- Data are collected retrospectively and elements of data may be missing or be of poor quality.

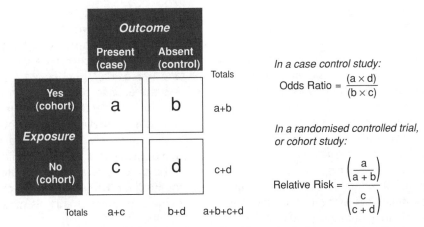

Figure 8.3 Contingency table illustrating the method for calculating an odds ratio or relative risk.

- Diseases that may cause acute mortality may result in the cases representing the survivors, which may lead to incorrect inferences such as the exposure factor being protective.
- Case-control studies may suffer from bias due to the method of selection of controls or the poor quality of recorded information or owner recall.

8.3.6 *Reporting the results of a case control study*

In a case control study the results are conventionally reported as an odds ratio. The calculation is relatively simple as shown in Fig. 8.3 because identical terms in the two odds (above and below the line) cancel out.

Odds Ratio, OR

$$= \frac{\text{odds of outcome in experimental group}}{\text{odds of outcome in control group}}$$

It is also possible to derive the Number Needed to Harm (NNH) from the OR and the Patients Experimental Event Rate (PEER, analogous to the experimental event rate described in section 9.5.15)

$$\text{NNH} = \frac{[\text{PEER} \times (\text{OR} - 1)] + 1}{[\text{PEER} \times (\text{OR} - 1)] \times (1 - \text{PEER})}$$

8.3.7 *Case-control examples*

The abstracts of two published case-control studies are presented below.

Diet and exercise as potential risk factors for osteochondritis dissecans in dogs (Slater et al., 1992)

A matched case-control study was conducted to evaluate dietary components and exercise patterns as potential risk factors for osteochondritis dissecans in dogs. A telephone interview, with a standard questionnaire and protocol, was used to collect data on dietary intake of calories and nutrients, and on the usual amounts and types of exercise of each dog. Thirty-one dogs with osteochondritis dissecans and 60 controls were matched on the basis of breed, sex, and age. Using a conditional logistic regression model, high dietary calcium, playing with other dogs, and drinking well water (rather than city water) were associated with increased risk of osteochondritis dissecans. Feeding of specialty dry dog foods was associated with decreased risk.

Comparison of medical and surgical treatment for impaction of the small colon in horses: 84 cases (1986–1996) (Rhoads et al., 1999).

Objective: To characterize clinical findings and compare effects of treatment and outcome for horses treated medically or surgically for impaction of the small colon. *Design*: Retrospective study. *Animals*: 84 horses with impaction of the small colon. *Procedure*: Medical records were reviewed for history, physical examination findings, laboratory values, treatment, response to treatment, complications, outcome, and necropsy findings. *Results*: 47 horses were treated medically and 37 horses were treated surgically. Significant differences between groups were not identified for duration of clinical signs, physical examination findings, or laboratory values. Horses treated surgically were hospitalised longer than horses treated medically. Complications recorded during hospitalisation included diarrhoea, jugular thrombophlebitis, recurrent colic, fever, and laminitis. Salmonella organisms were isolated from 20 horses. Horses treated surgically were more likely to have signs of moderate abdominal pain, gross abdominal distension, and positive results for culture of *Salmonella* spp than horses treated medically. Follow-up information was available for 27 horses treated medically and 23 horses treated surgically. Twenty-four (72%) and 21 (75%) of the horses, respectively, survived and were being used for their intended purpose at least 1 year after treatment. *Clinical implications*: Colitis may be a predisposing factor for impaction of the small colon in horses. Prognosis for horses treated surgically or medically is fair.

8.3.8   Case-control study design checklist

Is it an appropriate study for the scientific question?

This study design is often used to demonstrate associations between suspected causes and disease.

1. How are the cases to be selected?
2. Is there a clear case definition?
3. Has the target population been defined by the population of origin (general, specialist clinic?)

4. How are the control subjects to be obtained? Is the group from the same population as the comparison group? Are the two groups matched with regard to sex, age, breed, etc.?
5. Are the data to be collected in the same way for cases and controls? The information that is retrieved by owner interview or case note review must be standardized to avoid bias. Data collection techniques need to be critically reviewed to ensure they are identical for the two groups. Recall bias by owners of affected animals may bias the results.
6. Were there equal opportunities for exposure for members of case and control groups?
7. Can the design measure a dose-response effect?
8. Is the design appropriate to the aims? Often used to investigate possible cause and effect but is more appropriate for hypothesis generating.
9. Are there sufficient numbers of subjects?
10. Have the power and sample size been determined statistically?
11. Where are the potential biases and have these been addressed? This study design is very susceptible to sampling and measurement bias.
12. Could there be confounding factors? Beware that the association reported may be due to a third factor.
13. How will the results be statistically analysed?

8.4   Clinical questions and observational designs

Observational designs have the disadvantage when compared with clinical trials of being susceptible to the influence of the confounding variable.

Table 8.1 presents a comparison of the different observational designs and the parameters that

Table 8.1 Comparison of observational study designs.

Design	Advantages	Disadvantages	Parameters
Cohort, all	Establishes sequence of events Can study several outcomes Number of outcome events increases over time	Often requires large sample sizes Poor design for rare outcomes	Incidence Relative risk
Cohort, prospective	More control over selection of subjects More control over measurements Avoids bias in measuring variables	More expensive Longer duration	Incidence Relative risk
Cohort, retrospective	Less expensive Shorter duration	Less control over selection of subjects Less control over measurements	Incidence Relative risk
Cohort, multiple	Useful to investigate rare exposures or cohorts that have different exposures	Bias and confounding may increase	Incidence Relative risk
Cross-sectional	Can investigate several outcomes Study is of short duration Useful preliminary for a cohort study	Time sequence of exposure and outcome not established Inappropriate for rare outcomes and risk factors Incidence and true relative prevalence not established	Prevalence
Case-control	Appropriate design to study rare conditions Short study time Inexpensive Small scale	Potential for bias and confounding May not be able to establish time sequence of exposure to potential risk factor and outcome	Odds ratio (approximation of relative risk unless the outcome is common)
Nested-case control	All the advantages of a retrospective cohort design but with increased efficiency	Usually need to store samples until the outcome is known	Incidence Relative risk
Nested-case cohort	Use of a single control group for different case studies		

Source: Adapted from Hulley et al. (2007).

Table 8.2   Matching categories of clinical questions with study design.

Clinical question category	Design
Diagnosis (tests)	Cross-sectional, case-control
Prevalence	Cross-sectional
Incidence	Cohort
Risk	Cohort
	Case-control
Prognosis	Cohort
Treatment	Clinical trial
Prevention	Clinical trial
Cause	Cohort
	Case-control

Source: Adapted from Fletcher et al. (1996).

they can generate. Table 8.2 indicates the most appropriate designs to measure different categories of clinical questions.

8.5   Summary

1. Data collected in a cross-sectional study are measured at a single point in time, with no fundamental distinction between predictor variables and outcome variables. Cross-sectional studies provide valuable descriptions of prevalence.
2. Cross-sectional studies avoid the time, costs and dropout problems of follow-up designs.
3. Cross-sectional studies provide poor evidence for cause when compared to cohort studies, as the predictor variable cannot be proved to precede the outcome measure.
4. Cross-sectional studies need a large sample size, as compared with that required for a case-control study, when studying the prevalence of uncommon diseases and variables in the whole population.
5. In a case-control study, the prevalence of risk factors in a sample of animals that have a disease or other outcome of interest (cases) is compared with that in a sample of animals that do not (controls). Case-control studies, in which animals with and without the disease are sampled separately, is relatively inexpensive and provides the best method for studying uncommon diseases.
6. Sampling bias may be a major problem with case-control studies. The occurrence of sampling bias can be reduced by matching the cases and controls or the use of more than one control group, sampled using different methods.
7. Another potential problem with case-control studies is their retrospective design, which may result in measurement bias between the groups of cases and controls. This bias may be reduced by obtaining earlier measurements of the predictor variable and the use of blinding of the observers collecting or analysing the data.

8.6   References

Davies PR, Morrow WE, Miller DC, Deen J (1996) Epidemiological study of decubital ulcers in sows. *J. Am. Vet. Med. Assoc.* **208**(7): 1058–62.

Fletcher RH, Fletcher SW, Wagner EH (1996) Summing up. In: *Clinical Epidemiology (The Essentials)*, 3rd edn, Williams and Wilkins, Baltimore, p 255.

Hulley SB, Cummings SR, Browner WS, Grady DG, Newman TB (2007) Designing cross section and case studies. In: *Designing Clinical Research*, 3rd edn, Lippincott Williams and Wilkins, Philadelphia, pp 109–121.

Rhoads WS, Barton MH, Parks AH (1999) Comparison of medical and surgical treatment for impaction of the small colon in horses. *J. Am. Vet. Med. Assoc.* **214**(7): 1042–7.

Rose N, Larour G, Le Diguerher G, Eveno E, Jolly JP, Blanchard P, Oger A, Le Dimna M, Jestin A, Madec F (2003) Risk factors for porcine post-weaning multisystemic wasting syndrome (PMWS) in 149 French farrow-to-finish herds. *Prev. Vet. Med.* **61**(3): 209–25.

Slater MR, Scarlett JM, Donoghue S, Kaderly RE, Bonnett BN, Cockshutt J, Erb HN (1992) Diet and exercise as potential risk factors for osteochondritis dissecans in dogs. *Am. J. Vet. Res.* **53**(11): 2119–24.

8.7   Further reading

Ajetunmobi O (2002) Critical appraisal of retrospective studies. In: *Making Sense of Critical Appraisal*, Arnold, London, pp 112–21.

Dahoo IR, Waltner-Toews D (1985) Interpreting Clinical Research: Part I. General Considerations. *Compendium of Continuing Education* **7**(9): S474–S477.

Dahoo IR, Waltner-Toews D (1985) Interpreting Clinical Research: Part II. Descriptive and Experimental Studies. *Compendium of Continuing Education* **7**(9): S513–S519.

Dahoo IR, Waltner-Toews D (1985) Interpreting Clinical Research: Part 3 Observational Studies and Interpretation of Results. *Compendium of Continuing Education* **7**(9): S605–S613.

Fletcher RH, Fletcher SW, Wagner EH (1996) Studying cases. In: *Clinical Epidemiology (The Essentials)*, 3rd edn, Williams and Wilkins, Baltimore, pp 208–27.

Hulley SB, Newman TB, Cummings SR (2001) Designing an observational study. In: *Designing Clinical Research*, 2nd edn, Lippincott Williams and Wilkins, Philadelphia, pp 95–105.

Smith RD (2006) Risk assessment and prevention. In: *Veterinary Clinical Epidemiology*, 3rd edn, CRC Press, London, pp 91–109.

Thrusfield M (2005) Observational studies. In: *Veterinary Epidemiology*, 3rd edn, Blackwell Publishing, Oxford, pp 266–88.

Woodward M (2005) Case-control studies. In: *Epidemiology: Study and Data Analysis*, Chapman and Hall/CRC, London, pp 273–334.

8.8   MCQs

1 *In cross-sectional studies:*

(a) the variables are all measured at a single point in time
(b) the variables are measured going forwards in time
(c) the variables are measured going backwards in time
(d) no variables can be measured
(e) outcomes are not used.

2 *In prospective cohort studies:*

(a) the variables are all measured at a single point in time
(b) the variables are measured going forwards in time
(c) the variables are measured going backwards in time
(d) no variables can be measured
(e) outcomes are not used.

3 *In retrospective cohort studies:*

(a) the variables are all measured at a single point in time
(b) the variables are measured going forwards in time
(c) the variables are measured going backwards in time
(d) no variables can be measured
(e) outcomes are not used.

4 *In case-control studies:*

(a) the variables are all measured at a single point in time
(b) the variables are measured going forwards in time
(c) the variables are measured going backwards in time
(d) no variables can be measured
(e) outcomes are not used.

5 *Incidence can be measured using:*

(a) cross-sectional studies
(b) cohort studies
(c) case-control studies
(d) randomized controlled trials
(e) meta-analyses.

6 *The design providing the strongest evidence about causation is:*

(a) cross-sectional studies
(b) cohort studies
(c) case-control studies
(d) randomized controlled trials
(e) meta-analyses.

7 *The most appropriate design to study potential risk factors in rare diseases is:*

(a) cross-sectional studies
(b) cohort studies
(c) case-control studies
(d) randomized controlled trials
(e) meta-analyses.

8 *Matching in case-control studies:*

(a)   makes sampling easier
(b)   reduces sampling bias
(c)   reduces the cost of the study
(d)   reduces the size of the control group
(e)   reduces the number of variable measurements that need to be made.

9 *Stored samples from subjects in a nested case-control study:*

(a)   enable selective testing of the cohort once the outcomes are known
(b)   enable all the cohort to be batch tested
(c)   provide a reference base line
(d)   remove the need for further measurements
(e)   reduce confounding.

10 *Measurement bias can be reduced in case-control studies by:*

(a)   matching
(b)   blinding the owners and observers
(c)   using the same observer throughout the study
(d)   ensuring the observer knows the putative risk factor in the study
(e)   ensuring the observer knows whether the records are cases or controls.

8.9   MCQ answers

1. (a); 2. (b); 3. (c); 4. (c); 5. (b); 6. (b); 7. (c); 8. (b); 9. (a); 10. (b)

9

CLINICAL RANDOMIZED CONTROLLED TRIALS

Objectives

After reading this chapter readers should:

- understand the advantages and disadvantages of randomized controlled trials
- be able to recognize when an randomized controlled trial design is appropriate
- be able to plan and implement a randomized controlled trial.

9.1   Introduction

Clinical trials using a randomized controlled design have an important place amongst observational studies (cohort, case-control and cross-sectional studies) and in laboratory experiments. Randomized clinical controlled trials test hypotheses concerning a treatment or intervention that might be used on patients with disease; in contrast, retrospective and prospective cohort studies are generally used to test hypotheses about disease risk factors or prognosis.

In clinical trials, sometimes known as field trials, the subjects are left in their normal environment with the investigator controlling entry into the trial and the allocation to the treatment groups. The investigator does not control the exposure to disease or risk. Clinical trials are performed to evaluate the efficiency of an intervention in a real world setting. When properly designed they are considered to provide one of the most valid sources of evidence regarding a clinical question. They provide the most powerful designs for controlling the influence of confounding variables, and in establishing causality. Clinical trials are usually performed to evaluate therapeutic products or practices including vaccines, anthelmintics, antibiotics, analgesic drugs and management interventions. Clinical trials are usually performed at phase 3 in pharmaceutical development trials. They are relatively time-consuming and expensive to perform so they are often only undertaken when existing evidence suggests that a potential useful effect is likely to exist. These trials usually form part of the later stages of drug development and represent the

final hurdle before provisional approval is given for their use by the regulatory body. Phase 4 consists of an intensive monitoring period to identify potential adverse effects and provide further evidence of effectiveness in clinical practice.

Randomized controlled clinical trials should have a clearly defined research question and assess a clinically relevant outcome variable. They should use an appropriate study design and sample size for the question being asked. The design should include random assignment of animals to treatment and control groups, and a blinded assessment of the clinical outcome variable. The analysis of results should employ appropriate statistical analysis. These features are described and discussed below.

9.2   Randomized controlled trials

Randomized controlled trials may be experimental laboratory studies or experimental clinical trials. Experimental laboratory studies use experimental animals and reduce the variables by controlling the environment. The subjects may be artificially diseased (e.g. inoculated with an infectious pathogen) or a healthy population (e.g. in nutrition trials). The researcher has control over the allocation of animals into the groups being compared and control over the administration of the treatments to these groups. This method provides the best evidence of cause or treatment effect. However, the results may lack relevance to the real world due to the artificial environment.

Experimental clinical trials use animals that are kept in their normal environment. Any disease in the animal will have occurred naturally. Animals are usually allocated by the researcher to the treatment groups. If the protocols are well designed and performed properly, clinical trials provide the best evidence for the outcome that can be expected if the intervention is adopted for use in a population under field conditions.

A randomized controlled trial has two important features (Fig. 9.1).

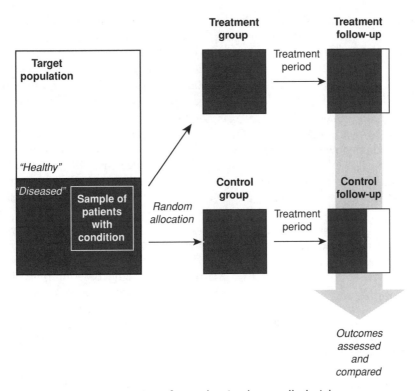

Figure 9.1 A schematic representation of a randomized controlled trial.

1. There are at least two groups, one or more treatment groups, and a control group
    The treatment group receives the treatment or intervention under investigation and the control group receives either no treatment or a standard default. The standard default contains all the ingredients at the same concentrations as the treatment but does not contain the active ingredient under investigation. This also acts as a placebo so that the owner does not know if their animal is in the treatment or the control group. The use of an established treatment may provide an alternative to a negative control when a failure to treat would be considered ethically unacceptable.
2. Patients are randomly assigned to the two groups. The two groups are observed in an identical fashion. The groups are followed for a specific length of time, at which point the

trial ends. Any differences in the trial outcome are attributable to the trial. Double blinding should be used if possible. A trial in which neither the owner/animal nor the veterinary surgeon knows which treatment the animal is receiving is called double blind. This avoids bias. The measured outcome therefore relates to the actual treatment not the act of giving a treatment.

The control group allows a comparison to be made between the treatment (intervention) and a chosen alternative, such as no treatment or an alternative therapy. This is important as an excellent cure rate without a control may simply reflect the outcome of the natural course of the disease irrespective of the treatment used. The two groups are compared prospectively for the disease or other outcomes of interest.

The randomized controlled trial is the design of choice for answering questions about the effectiveness of different treatments.

9.2.1 Advantages

- Random allocation reduces the risk of bias and is the most powerful method of eliminating known and unknown confounding variables.
- The allocation of subjects, and the number of subjects, to treatments is planned.
- Cause precedes effect.
- It increases the probability that the differences between the groups can be attributed to the treatment.

9.2.2 Disadvantages

- Sometimes it is unethical to allow for an untreated control group due to the severity of the effects of withholding an effective treatment.
- These studies are expensive to conduct and relatively rare in veterinary medicine.

9.2.3 Examples

Effect of perioperative prophylactic antimicrobial treatment in dogs undergoing elective orthopaedic surgery (Whittem et al., 1999)

Objective: To determine whether perioperative antimicrobial prophylaxis would reduce incidence of postoperative infection among dogs undergoing elective orthopaedic procedures. *Design*: Randomised, controlled, blinded, intention clinical trial. *Animals*: Dogs of any breed, sex, or age undergoing elective orthopaedic surgery at a veterinary teaching hospital. *Procedures*: Dogs were randomly assigned to 1 of 3 groups: treatment with saline solution, treatment with potassium penicillin G and treatment with cefazolin. Treatments were intended to be administered within 30 minutes prior to surgery; a second dose was administered if

surgery lasted > 90 minutes. Dogs were monitored for 10 to 14 days after surgery for evidence of infection. *Results*: After the first 112 dogs were enrolled in the study, it was found that infection rate for control dogs (5/32 dogs) was significantly higher than the rate for dogs treated with antimicrobials (3/80 dogs). Therefore, no more dogs were enrolled in the study. A total of 126 dogs completed the study. Monte Carlo simulations indicated that compared with dogs that received antimicrobials prophylactically, dogs that received saline solution developed infections significantly more frequently. Difference in efficacy, however, was not observed between the 2 antimicrobial drugs used. *Conclusions and clinical relevance*: Results indicated that perioperative antimicrobial prophylaxis decreased postoperative infection rate in dogs undergoing elective orthopaedic surgery, compared with infection rate in control dogs. Cefazolin was not more efficacious than potassium penicillin G in these dogs.

Controlled clinical trial of the effect of a homoeopathic nosode on the somatic cell counts in the milk of clinically normal dairy cows (Holmes et al., 2005)

Cows in a 250-cow Holstein–Friesian herd were allocated at random to be treated with either a homoeopathic nosode or a negative control, both treatments being applied by means of an aerosol spray to the vulval mucous membranes. A total of six treatments were given over a period of three days and milk samples were taken for the determination of somatic cell counts (SCC) on days -3, 3, 7, 9, 14, 21 and 28. Individuals applying the treatments or carrying out the SCC determination were unaware of which animals were receiving which treatment. Owing to the wide natural variations in SCC, the trial had only a 71 per cent possibility of detecting a 30 per cent difference in SCC between the two groups. There were no significant differences between the SCC of the two groups on any sample day, but there were significant variations between the SCC on different days ($P = 0.003$) in both groups.

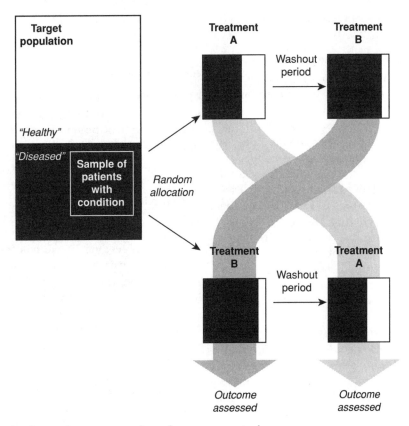

Figure 9.2 A schematic representation of a crossover study.

9.3 Cross-over designs

A sample population is randomly assigned to one of two treatment groups and followed over time to see if they develop the outcome of interest. After a period of time during which the outcome would have been expected to occur they are switched to the other treatment, sometimes with a washout period in between (Fig. 9.2). They are then monitored for a further period and the outcomes during this period noted.

9.3.1 Advantages

- Because the subjects act as their own control the number of animals can usually be reduced compared to a randomized controlled trial.

9.3.2 Disadvantages

- Treatments with persistent actions confound the results.
- Cross-over studies are suitable only for long-term conditions for which treatment provides only short-term relief, e.g. chronic arthritis.
- The trial period has a long duration (at least twice as long as parallel studies) and a higher chance of drop out before follow-up.
- There is increased complexity for the owners and in the analysis of results.

9.3.3 Example

Effects of insoluble and soluble dietary fiber on glycemic control in dogs with naturally

occurring insulin-dependent diabetes mellitus (Kimmel et al., 2000)

Objective: To evaluate the effects of diets differing in type and quantity of fiber on glycemic control in dogs with naturally occurring insulin-dependent diabetes mellitus. *Design*: Prospective randomized crossover controlled trial. *Animals*: 7 dogs with well-regulated naturally occurring insulin-dependent diabetes mellitus. *Procedure*: Dogs were fed 1 of 3 diets for 1 month each in 1 of 6 randomized diet sequences. Diets included a low-fiber diet (LF) and 2 high-fiber diets; 1 contained only insoluble fiber (HIF), and 1 contained soluble fiber in addition to insoluble fiber (HSF). Caloric intake was unchanged throughout the study. Glycemic control was assessed after each feeding trial by measuring serum fructosamine concentration and performing 5 serial measurements of blood glucose concentration every 2 hours after the morning feeding and insulin injection. *Results*: Significant differences were not detected in body weight, required insulin dosage, or albumin concentration among dogs fed the HIF, HSF, and LF diets. Mean and maximum blood glucose concentrations and area under the blood glucose curve were significantly lower in dogs fed the HIF diet, compared with values in the same dogs fed the HSF or LF diet. Fructosamine concentration was significantly lower in dogs fed the HIF or HSF diet, compared with values in the same dogs fed the LF diet. *Conclusions and clinical relevance*: In dogs with naturally occurring insulin-dependent diabetes mellitus, a dry, high insoluble-fiber diet may aid in glycemic control.

9.4   Factorial design trials

Factorial designs can be used to investigate interactions between treatments or interventions. In the simplest design two interventions (A and B) are compared. All possible combinations of the two interventions are represented. The four groups are A Placebo B, B Placebo A, AB, Placebo A and Placebo B. The subjects are randomly allocated to one of the four groups. This is illustrated in Fig. 9.3. The factorial design can be expanded

to accommodate other factors, although the sample size will increase.

9.4.1   Example

Clinical efficacy of flunixin, carprofen and ketoprofen as adjuncts to the antibacterial treatment of bovine respiratory disease (Lockwood et al., 2003)

Three non-steroidal anti-inflammatory drugs (NSAIDs), flunixin, ketoprofen and carprofen, were used in conjunction with ceftiofur, in the treatment of naturally occurring bovine respiratory disease. Sixty-six mixed-breed beef cattle weighing on average 197 kg met the inclusion criteria of pyrexia of at least 40 degrees C, an illness score indicating at least moderate illness and at least moderate dyspnoea. They were allocated randomly to four treatment groups. All the groups received ceftiofur for three days at a dose rate of 1.1 mg/kg by intramuscular injection, and three groups received, in addition, a single dose of either flunixin (2.2 mg/kg by intravenous injection) or ketoprofen (3 mg/kg by intravenous injection) or carprofen (1.4 mg/kg by subcutaneous injection). During the first 24 hours of the study, the pyrexia of the three groups treated with a NSAID was reduced significantly more than the pyrexia of the group treated with ceftiofur alone, and two and four hours after treatment the reduction in pyrexia was significantly greater in the groups treated with flunixin and ketoprofen than in the group treated with carprofen. There were no statistically significant differences between the four groups with respect to depression, illness scores, dyspnoea or coughing. There was less lung consolidation in the three groups treated with a NSAID than in the animals treated with ceftiofur alone, but the difference was significant only in the group treated with flunixin.

9.5   Features of randomized clinical trials

The power and the validity of the study are dependent on a number of important design features of the study. Factors which may impact

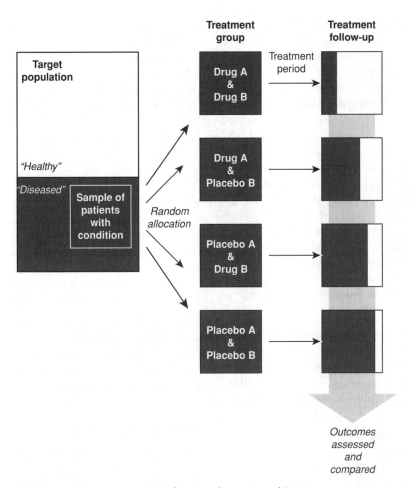

Figure 9.3 Factorial design investigating the two drugs, A and B.

on theses components are: blinding, randomization and analysis by intention to treat. Randomization avoids selection bias and blinding avoids observer bias. Bias may occur unless an intention-to-treat analysis is performed which includes all the subjects originally recruited into the group. Small size can result in bias due to random chance effects impacting on results. The duration, dose or intensity of treatment or observation period may be inadequate to demonstrate a difference.

9.5.1 Sample size

A power calculation should be performed to estimate the sample size required for a defined sta-

tistically significant difference before considering exclusion criteria. The estimation of sample size is extremely important to avoid studies with insufficient power. Consideration should be given to the possible consequences of participants who are lost to follow-up. The investigator should ensure there is a large accessible population and enough time and money to get the desired sample size once entry and exclusion criteria have been defined.

9.5.2 Selecting the participants

Entry and exclusion criteria for subjects from the target population need to be defined. It is a wise precaution to obtain consent before applying the criteria to ensure the subjects selected will participate. The entry criteria should maximize the primary outcome under investigation, the ease of recruitment, the effectiveness of the treatment, the generalizability of the results and the likelihood of compliance and follow-up. A balance may have to be struck between selecting the risk of outcome with the generalizability of the results. Time constraints, cost and sample size may necessitate the selection of subjects that represent a specialized target population. Initial screening of potential participants may be helpful in selecting subjects who will adhere to the protocol but care is needed not to introduce bias. Giving all potential participants a placebo for a trial period and closely measuring the compliance may identify unsuitable participants before randomization to the treatment and control groups.

Exclusion criteria should be defined after careful consideration of the impact on the generalizability of the results, the ability to recruit a sufficient number of subjects, and the increased cost and complexity of recruitment. Important criteria for exclusion are:

- Prior knowledge that a treatment may be unsafe or have an adverse side effect in a defined subset of the target population.
- Prior knowledge that allocation to the placebo group would adversely affect the progression of a disease.
- Subjects in whom the treatment is unlikely to have any beneficial effect.
- Subjects who are unlikely to comply with the treatment, recording of measurements or be available for follow-up.

This information may require informed consent to access patient records before or during the recruitment process.

9.5.3   *Measuring baseline variables of the trial subjects*

Owners' contact details must be recorded and informed consent obtained. Predefined check-

lists should be used to determine important patient characteristics, which will help to define how representative the subjects are of the proposed target population. This information will also be needed if a stratification design is anticipated. Baseline variables which are related to the primary and secondary hypotheses should be measured and recorded.

9.5.4   *Case criteria*

If the efficacy of a treatment is being tested for a specific disease it is essential that the subject entering the trial have the disease. Sometimes the treatment may be specifically targeted at a clinical stage in the severity of the disease. Clear clinical definitions or test results need to be defined as part of the entry criteria.

Similarly, if a preventative intervention is being studied it is vital that there is a clear definition of when a patient has developed the outcome. The frequency of systematic monitoring must be clearly stated in the protocol instructions.

9.5.5   *Randomization*

Owners need to complete the baseline evaluation and be found eligible for inclusion before allocation occurs. Randomization is used to ensure that patients are allocated to each intervention to exclude selection bias and balance the distribution of variables that may influence the outcome measures. The allocation when blinding is used needs to be tamper-proof and a statement at which point and who will reveal the groups needs to be indicated in the protocol; sealed envelopes are often used.

In general terms the preferred approach is to randomize equal numbers of participants to each group. However, depending on the number of treatments in the study, optimal study sizes for each group may differ. Trials with small study sizes will have a gain in power if specialized randomized procedures are used to balance the group sizes and variables. These techniques are called block randomization and stratified block randomization, respectively.

Simple randomization

This may involve tossing a coin or using computer-generated randomization to allocate subjects to treatment groups. If the trial is small then by chance the numbers allocated to each group can be uneven. Block randomization can avoid this problem.

Block randomization

Block randomization is a common technique that is used to ensure there are equal numbers of participants in each treatment group. In a trial using two treatments and 40 animals, the animals could be divided into blocks of four animals. There are six possible combinations in which two treatments can be given to four animals. If the treatments were A and B the combinations would be (1) AABB, (2) ABAB, (3) ABBA, (4) BBAA, (5) BAAB and (6) BABA. One of the six combinations is selected by using simple randomization methods and is allocated to the next four animals entering the trial. The next four animals are given the treatments in the sequence indicated by the selected combination.

Matched pairs randomization

This is another strategy for balancing baseline confounding variables where there are two treatment groups. Pairs of subjects are matched on important factors such as breed, age and sex, and then one member of the pair is randomly assigned to a treatment group and the matched pair is assigned to the other treatment group. This ensures equal group sizes.

Stratified randomization

The experimental population is stratified by possible confounding variables before randomizing the subjects within each stratum to the groups within the clinical trial. This ensures that the groups contain equal numbers of subjects from each stratum so the potential confounders are balanced between the groups.

Cluster randomized designs

In multicentre studies or studies using pens of animals the treatment centres themselves or pens and not individual subjects are randomized to the treatments. All the subjects in one centre receive the same treatment. This design can be useful when it is impossible to blind the veterinarian to the treatments.

Other allocation methods

Other allocation methods have been used, such as selecting every alternate animal entering a dairy parlour to create two treatment groups or allocating the animals to the groups based on the next available animal to enter the study. To limit the number of animals receiving the least effective treatment an allocation method called 'play the winner' has been used. The first subject entering the trial is allocated by simple randomization procedure. Every subsequent allocation is based on the success or failure of the immediate predecessor in the trial. If the treatment was a success the next subject gets the same treatment; if it was a failure then the next subject gets the alternative treatment. These methods should not be used when randomization is a viable alternative.

9.5.6   Blinding

Concealment, hiding the result of the random allocation from everyone involved in the trial, is another important component of randomization and is known as 'blinding'. Blinding can be used to minimize observer bias. It protects the trial from animals in different groups being handled differently and avoids biased assessment of outcomes. Logistically, blinding can be difficult to achieve as it may necessitate considerable effort to make the placebo physically and chemically similar to the treatment in all respects other than the active ingredient. Sometimes it is impossible to blind the trial if a physical procedure is under investigation. In these cases objective measures and clear detailed instructions regarding the measurements of the outcome variable are vital to obviate observer bias.

Single-blind means that the owner does not know which treatment has been given to their animal but the veterinarian does. In a trial where the owner has to provide information about their animal this is essential. In a double-blind trial neither the owner nor the veterinarian (investigator) knows which treatment has been given.

If the same investigator is used to assess the study groups it may become obvious to the investigator that one group has a characteristic outcome. Bias may then be introduced, as the investigator will assume knowledge of group identity with regard to the active treatments. Removing access to the interim results and using different investigators for different groups are possible strategies, although with subjective observations this may introduce another bias. Asking the investigator to identify the groups before they are revealed may provide an indicator for the potential of bias.

9.5.7   Treatments and types of comparison

Superiority trials

Most trials are superiority trials, where the intervention is tested against either an inactive therapy (placebo) or an active therapy. The aim of the trial is to show that the intervention is superior to the control. This type of trial has a null hypothesis stating that there is no difference between the test drug and the control in terms of a defined outcome variable and the alternative hypothesis stating that there is a difference.

A placebo-controlled superiority trial is usually used as the gold standard by regulatory authorities in the drug approval process where the effect of the test drug must exceed some prescribed threshold considered to be clinically relevant.

Equivalence trials

Equivalence trials aim to show that the effects of two active interventions do not differ by more than a specified amount in either direction. Bioequivalence trials measure the pharmacological dynamics to determine the therapeutic equivalence of two drugs.

Non-inferiority trials

Non-inferiority trials aim to show that an intervention is not worse than an active control by more than an equivalence margin.

Treatment factors to consider in trial design

- Effectiveness and safety.
- Feasibility of blinding.
- Number of treatments to be studied in the trial.
- Whether different dose rates will be studied.
- Sample population and the generalizability of the results.

If there are many uncertainties a pilot study may be a useful preliminary to refine a larger study. In drug development a wide range of doses, regimens and length of treatment may be studied in a series of clinical trials to establish the most acceptable in terms of safety and effectiveness for further evaluation. Effectiveness needs to be carefully considered in severe diseases and those with a high risk of mortality. When selecting a dose rate the highest tolerable dose may be the best choice. Safety should be the main consideration with diseases that are mild and have a low risk of mortality. The lowest effective dose may be the best choice for these patients. Trials with single interventions are easier to plan, manage and interpret. Consideration should be given to the ease of introduction into clinical practice when contemplating the route and frequency of medication so that the outcomes can be easily translated to general clinical practice.

9.5.8   Controls and placebos

The best controls use inactive placebos although ethics may preclude the withholding of treatment/prevention in a treatment trial. Placebos can be used to avoid any influence of the measurements of the variable caused by the administration of the intervention, or the changes in behaviour by the owner. The placebo replicates the administration method and content of the intervention with the exception of the active component.

If alternative treatments are used as a control in a trial the analysis will be required to demonstrate superiority of one treatment over another. The failure to demonstrate such superiority may not necessarily mean that there is no difference between the treatments where there is insufficient power. Equivalence trials, i.e. trials designed to demonstrate a lack of difference (or equivalence), require different sample size considerations and are sometimes performed to identify new treatments that have advantages other than effectiveness. These may include fewer side effects (greater safety), increased dosing intervals and lower cost. It is important to establish the power of such studies to ensure the interpretation is quantified.

9.5.9   Optimizing follow-up and protocol adherence

Adherence to the treatment protocols is essential if the study is to retain statistical power. Loss of study participant results in a reduction in the power of the study and weakens the evidence produced. If protocols are not adhered to then bias may be introduced, which will invalidate the conclusions. Besides the loss in power, bias can be introduced as a specific subgroup that experiences unpleasant side effects may be the participants that drop out. If animals are not treated then the outcomes will be affected.

There are many reasons for poor compliance and these should be carefully considered when designing instruction protocols, monitoring systems and recruiting subjects. Reasons for poor compliance may include lack of understanding of the instructions, confusion by the complexity of the treatment regimen, perceived side effects, the length of the trial, poor communication, lack of response, loss of interest and personal reasons for leaving the area. Compliance can be improved by careful selection of recruits, financial incentives, frequent communication with the study investigator, motivational visits and talks, a simple recording system, treatment prompts, simple instructions and reasonable time limits to the trial.

Enhancing adherence and reducing dropouts may be achieved by explaining the importance of the trial, expressing appreciation during the trial, using short duration trials, providing simple regimens, using prompts and appropriate labelling of medication. Simple measures that are painless and easily performed in a nearby clinic or at home will improve protocol adherence. Consistent interpersonal contact with the owners has a positive effect on participants.

Attempts should be made to monitor adherence by using report cards or auditing the pills used. Ensuring contact details are correct is vital to optimize communication.

Even if the participants do not adhere to the protocol or discontinue the trial intervention they should be followed so that their outcomes can be included in the intention-to-treat analysis and a conservative but valid result obtained.

9.5.10   Measuring outcome and adverse effects

Clinical relevance, feasibility and cost need to be carefully considered when deciding on the outcome variables to measure. Indirect variables of an outcome are sometimes known as surrogate markers. Surrogate markers must be biologically plausible and strongly associated with and specific to the outcome of interest. Creatinine phosphokinase levels, as an indicator of muscle damage, are an example. The outcome variable should be one that can be measured accurately and precisely. Continuous measures of outcome variables have greater power than other measurement categories. It is often desirable to record several outcome variables that measure different components of the phenomena of interest. Subjective measures need to be defined and described in detail. The study should include measurements that are associated with known side/adverse effects. In the early trials a very broad approach may be taken to detect unknown side/adverse effects by monitoring a wide range of variables. Expense in larger later trials usually means that these variables are reduced. The sample size and the end point for adverse effects in a study design may be different from those for investigating benefits and investigators should be aware of this. Rare side effects may only become apparent once the drug is in widespread clinical usage.

9.5.11   Terminating trials

In the protocol it is important to have a decision rule which indicates the termination of the trial should severe adverse side effects occur. In open trials using interim analysis a termination point will be indicated by a predetermined level of significance.

9.5.12   Intention-to-treat analysis

This analysis is recommended for all randomized controlled trials. Participants (the owners or keepers of the animals) who choose not to use some or all of the assigned interventions are included in the estimates of the effects of that intervention. This approach hedges on the side of caution when interpreting the data but provides a realistic assessment of the overall cost of treatment and benefit to the entire population.

9.5.13   Monitoring clinical trials

Investigators must ensure that participants are not exposed to a harmful intervention, denied a beneficial intervention or continue in a trial that cannot answer the research question. Interim analyses of results are useful to monitor for these situations. The protocol should indicate how these issues will be monitored, the benchmarks to be used and the actions to be taken.

9.5.14   Analyses

The results of clinical randomized controlled trials are usually parameterized using some of the following measures:

- odds ratio (OR)
- relative risk reduction (RRR)
- absolute risk reduction (ARR)
- relative benefit
- absolute benefit
- number needed to treat/harm (NNT/NNH)
- *P* values
- confidence intervals

It is important that careful consideration is given to the values being measured and how the data will be statistically analysed to optimize the clinical relevance.

Analyses of trial results are performed at predetermined time points before the end of the trial. This enables significantly beneficial or harmful side effects to be identified as early as possible. Because of the dangers of a type I error (false positive) the *P* value in the early stages of an interim analysis should be set at a more stringent level, e.g. $P < 0.01$ as opposed to $P < 0.05$. In open trials the study continues until a desired level of significance is reached. In closed trials the trial is terminated if a specified difference is not reached by a defined end point, which may be based on the time or number of subjects.

The main outcomes of randomized controlled trials are likely to include the proportion of animals showing a beneficial treatment effect and the proportion of animals developing adverse reactions. These are called event rates (see Fig. 9.4).

The **control event rate** (CER) is the proportion of animals in the control group (either placebo, or a

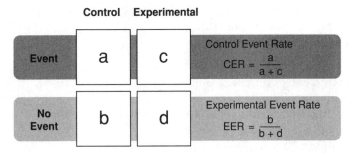

Figure 9.4 Contingency table illustrating the method for calculating control event rates and experimental event rates.

non-experimental treatment) demonstrating an effect.

The **experimental event rate** (EER) is the proportion of animals receiving the test treatment demonstrating an effect.

Relative Risk Reduction (RRR)

Relative risk reduction is the proportion by which the treated group improves compared to the control group.

$$RRR = \frac{CER - EER}{CER}$$

Absolute Risk Reduction (ARR)

Absolute risk reduction is the absolute difference between the control and experimental group.

$$ARR = CER - EER$$

ARR is a more useful measure in most clinical situations. RRR removes consideration of the background risk so that when looking at a rare event a small difference in the treatment group produces the same RRR as a large difference when looking at a more common event.

Consider two different clinical situations, two different diseases for which vaccination is effective. In the first disease 88% of unvaccinated animals develop the disease, and 15% of vaccinates. In the second disease in which 8.8% of unvaccinated animals develop the disease which is reduced to 1.5% on vaccination (Table 9.1).

The two vaccines against the different diseases have identical relative risk reductions but the absolute benefits have a ten-fold difference.

Number needed to treat (NNT)

An extremely useful measure of benefit, which most of us find easy to understand is the inverse of the absolute risk reduction. It tells us the number of patients we would have to treat in order to prevent one bad outcome.

$$NNT = \frac{1}{ARR}$$

Table 9.1 Two different diseases for which vaccination is effective.

	CER (un-vaccinated)	EER (vaccinated)	ARR	RRR
Disease 1	0.88 (88%)	.15 (15%)	0.88 − 0.15 = 0.73 (73%)	$\frac{0.88 - 0.15}{0.88} = 83\%$
Disease 2	0.088 (8.8%)	0.015 (1.5%)	0.088 − 0.015 = 0.073 (7%)	$\frac{0.088 - 0.015}{0.088} = 83\%$

Similarly an increase in adverse outcomes is described as a 'number needed to harm' (NNH) which would otherwise be a negative NNT value.

In a paper by Olivry et al. (2002) the use of oral cyclosporine was compared to the use of prednisolone for the treatment of canine atopic dermatitis in a randomised controlled trial. In the results of the trial it was reported that there was a reduction in pruritus in 71% (10/14) of dogs treated with prednisolone and in 77% (10/13) of dogs treated with cyclosporine. The ARR of prorates resulting from the use of cyclosporine was 0.06 (77%–71%).

Therefore the NNT in order to achieve the relief of pruritus in one extra case is:

$$NNT = \frac{1}{0.06} = 16.7 \approx 17 \text{ dogs}$$

Confidence intervals (CIs)

The usefulness of confidence intervals is their ability to set single values in perspective. A NNT of 7 with a 95% CI of 3 to 9 is clearly more useful than a NNT of 7 with a 95% CI of 3 to 28.

95% CI on the ARR

$$= \pm 1.96 \times \sqrt{\frac{CER \times (1 - CER)}{\# \text{ of control animals}} + \frac{EER \times (1 - EER)}{\# \text{ of exper. animals}}}$$

If we apply this to the clinical trial results used as an example above we would calculate the following 95% CI for the ARR:

95% CI on the ARR

$$= \pm 1.96 \times \sqrt{\frac{0.71 \times (1 - 0.71)}{14} + \frac{0.77 \times (1 - 0.77)}{13}}$$

95% CI on the ARR

$$= \pm 1.96 \times 0.168 = \pm 0.33 \text{ or } 33\%$$

Clearly the confidence intervals on the risk reduction are greater than the risk reduction itself and so we are forced to conclude that the evidence for using cyclophosphamide over prednisolone is unproven in the results from this trial (the small

group sizes was the problem in this case).

The 95% CI on an NNT = 1/the 95% CI on its ARR.

When a confidence crosses the line of no difference (i.e. the point at which it becomes disadvantageous), then we can conclude that the results are not clinically useful.

9.5.15 *Design and implementation factors checklist*

1. Does the study ask a clearly focused question?
   Is the population clearly described?
   Is the intervention clearly stated?
   Is the outcome to be measured clearly stated?
2. Is this study design appropriate to answer the question?
3. Will the animals be appropriately allocated to intervention (treatment) and control groups? Will the subjects be randomly allocated to treatment and control groups and should there be matching or stratification?
4. Will the owners/researchers be blinded to the study animals? Were the observers (e.g. owners, clinicians, researchers, technicians) blinded (masked) to the subject's group allocation?
5. Has a sample size calculation been performed? Will the number of animals used be large enough to ensure the power of the experiment will indicate a meaningful difference?
6. Are protocols in place to monitor and keep track of all the animals that entered the trial?
7. Will both groups be treated equally other than the intervention?
8. Are the chosen outcome measures appropriate?
9. Will all the animals in all the groups be followed up and data collected in the same way? Will all subjects be examined with equal intensity and will the observers doing the measurements be blinded?

10. Which statistical tests will be used to analyse the results?
11. Will confidence intervals be provided?
12. Will side effects be recorded? The beneficial effect of any therapy has to be balanced against its side effects. Often the therapeutics effect far outweighs the adverse effect. But when two similar treatments are being compared, a difference in side effects could be more important than the treatment difference.
13. Did an ethics committee approve the trial?

9.6 Poorly controlled or uncontrolled trials

9.6.1 Comparisons between groups at different times

Historical data from subjects that did not receive the treatment are used for comparison with the current experimental group. Historical controls often have poor outcomes and are rarely matched appropriately to the current treatment group. As a consequence these comparisons often show the test treatment in a favourable light and should be viewed with caution, as there are many other variables that may have affected the result.

9.6.2 Comparisons between different places

If league tables of performance and outcomes were introduced into the veterinary profession as a means of auditing competency there would be a grave danger that, in the absence of a detailed demographic analysis, the results would be misinterpreted. These tables may be able to highlight areas of potential concern, but without more detailed scientific validation the evidence supplied by such information is usually weak.

9.6.3 n = 1 trials (the 'treat and see' method)

All veterinary surgeons have used the 'treat and see' approach as a valid methodology in the treatment of individual patients. A good example is the treatment of osteoarthritis in the aging dog, where there is a wide selection of treatment options. Although evidence is available in the literature, individual patient circumstances and variation in response sometimes mean that the best treatment is not always obvious. In order to select the best treatment for an individual patient a trial of different therapies used sequentially is performed on the animal in question. In order to increase the objectivity of this exercise, good patient records, using well-defined descriptors, should be used to identify the best treatment, rather than relying on memory.

9.6.4 Uncontrolled trials ('before and after' trials)

Some trials evaluate outcomes before and after an intervention has been introduced, and assume that the difference between them is solely due the intervention. This is a dangerous assumption as there are many factors that are time dependent.

Another form of uncontrolled study presents the outcomes and harm from a cohort of treated patients. This study cannot distinguish between the outcome with the treatment and without the treatment, as the observations may just reflect the natural history of the disease rather than any effect of the treatment.

9.6.5 Non-random allocation trials

Bias is a major problem with non-randomized trials. True randomization involves the use of a formal randomizing method and should not be confused with the arbitrary assignment of animals to treatments. Selecting alternate cases for treatments or using a different treatment on certain days of the week are examples of arbitrary selection and may introduce confounding factors, however unlikely it may seem. True randomization is extremely easy to achieve and is only avoided as a result of ignorance or laziness.

9.7   Protocols

Trial protocols are required by the regulatory authorities if the trial forms part of the licensing data. This enables a systematic assessment of the validity and the efficacy of the drug to be made. Detailed protocols should be produced for any clinical trial to document the proposed design, methods and results analysis. The protocol serves two main functions: it is the justification for the study, which will be scrutinized by the ethics committee, and it is a reference manual for all those involved in the study.

Woodward (2005) produced the following general principles for the protocol:

1. Rationale: The background to the study. When a novel treatment is involved, this might include an explanation of how it is thought to work against the disease in question and why it might be an improvement on existing treatment. References to previous literature on the subject would normally be included.
2. Aims of study: What, exactly, does the study seek to discover? For instance, the aims may be to compare the efficacy (suitably defined) and side effects of a new treatment against an existing treatment.
3. Design of study: A specification of the basic design used and how the measures to avoid bias will be implemented.
4. Selection of subjects: This should include the number to be assigned to each treatment group, as well as inclusion and exclusion criteria. Inclusion criteria usually contain the precise definition of the disease to be used (for example, the signs that must be exhibited) and appropriate age limits (if any) for entry to the study. Exclusion criteria often include other medical conditions that may cause complications, and

pregnancy. Subjects may also be excluded because they have received treatment that may affect their responses in the current investigation.
5. Drugs and dosages: A list of the medications (or alternatives) to be taken by the subjects, the dosage(s) to be used and the form of the medication (tablets, injections, inhalers, etc.). The drug supplier is mentioned here if not specified elsewhere.
6. Assessments: What the study will measure. This is likely to include measures of efficacy, records of adverse events plus records of compliance (how many tablets were actually taken each day) and concurrent medication (or other form of treatment) received. Compliance gives important information on tolerance of treatment and treatment administration. Records of concurrent medication may be used in two main ways. If this medication is something that alleviates the symptoms of the very disease being studied, then its consumption is evidence of lack of efficacy of the treatment allocated. If the medication is normally taken for other complaints, then its consumption might indicate a side effect of the treatment allocated. Furthermore, in the event that many subjects take the same concurrent medication, we may wish to look at the effect of taking a combination of the study treatment and the concurrent medication.
7. Documentation: A list of the forms for recording information. This may include physicians' record cards to be completed during clinic visits and daily record cards to be completed by the subject. The latter would typically record compliance and side effects, plus self-assessments of well-being (particularly in studies of chronic conditions).
8. Procedure: Usually the longest part of the protocol, this specifies what should be done, and by whom, at each stage of the study. Many intervention studies

involve several clinic visits and here we should state, for example, what measurements will be taken at each particular visit, including the precise methodology to use. Instructions for the doctor to give to her or his patients would also be included (such as how many tablets should be taken per day and how the daily record card should be completed).

9. Withdrawals: Subjects may withdraw or be removed from the study by the investigating physician (or others), possibly for medical reasons or because of serious protocol deviations. This section of the protocol specifies how the reasons for withdrawal should be recorded (often on a special form) and describes any other consequent administrative procedures. Reasons for withdrawal may, of course, provide evidence of side effects.

10. Adverse events: As for withdrawals. Severe adverse events would often lead to withdrawal in any case.

11. Consent: A statement that subject consent (or a proxy, if necessary) will be sought and how this will be obtained.

12. Ethics: A statement that the appropriate ethical committee will be, or has already been, consulted. A copy of the ethical guidelines to be adopted, such as the Declaration of Helsinki, is often included as an appendix.

13. Analysis: Outline details (at least) of the statistical methods to be used on the subsequent data set. If there are special features of the required analysis, such as separate subgroup analyses (for example, by age group), these should be given here.

14. Data discharge: Details of data confidentiality and the rules governing disclosure.

15. Investigators' statement: A declaration that the protocol will be followed, which the principal investigators (and others) will sign.

Table 9.2 and 9.3 provide checklists for randomized controlled trials.

9.8 Summary

1. A RCT is the most powerful study design for eliminating the effects of confounding variables when investigating interventions.
2. Inclusion and exclusion criteria must be explicit.
3. The sample must represent the target population.
4. Informed consent is essential.
5. The sample must be randomly allocated to two or more groups.
6. Stratification and matching can be used to reduce the impact of chance uneven distribution of potentially confounding variables.
7. Base line values for outcome variables must be recorded at the start of the trial.
8. Bias will be reduced by blinding the owners and the investigators.
9. If an untreated control group is used a placebo should be used to demonstrate any observed difference is due to the proposed active component of the treatment.
10. Protocols indicating the frequency, timing and dose rate need to be clearly defined.
11. Outcome variables should be chosen that have a strong association with the phenomena of interest and which can be accurately measured.
12. Monitoring for adverse effects and defined endpoints regarding the severity of disease and poor responses must be included in the study protocol.
13. Interim results analysis may enable the trial to be shortened.
14. It is essential that treatment compliance is maximised (validity maintained) and dropout rates are minimised (power maintained).
15. Intention to treat analysis should be performed so that the outcomes are not overestimated.

Table 9.2   Checklist of components for a clinical trial (modified from Noordhuizen et al. (1993) and Thrusfield (2005)).

General information
   Title of trial
   Names and addresses of investigator and sponsors
   Identity of trial sites
Justification and objectives
   Reasons for trial
   Hypothesis to be tested
   Primary end point
Design
   Variables to be measured
   Measures to be used
   Power of experiment
Duration
   Period and dates of trial
   Time frame for recruitment of cases
   Course of clinical disease under investigation
   Duration of treatment and withdrawal periods (farm animals)
   Decision rules for terminating e.g. clinical severity
Study population
   The subjects
   Inclusion/exclusion criteria
   Case definition/diagnostic criteria
   Selection of controls
   Identification of individuals within groups
   Sample size computation
   Owner's informed consent
Intervention
   Dosage/vaccine regime/procedure
   Product description
   Method of administration
   Placebo description and method of administration
   Operator's safety protocols
   Blinding methods
   Compliance monitoring and recording
Type of trial
   Method of subject allocation
   Stratification variables
Data collection
   Data to be collected and recording system
   Frequency and method of data collection
   Recording system for adverse reactions
   Training
   Confidentiality requirement
Data analysis
   Unblinding protocol
   Statistical methods to be used
   Description of how withdrawals and animals lost to follow-up will be analysed

Table 9.3 CONSORT* checklist of items to include when reporting a randomized trial.

Paper section and topic	Description
Title and abstract	How participants were allocated to interventions (e.g. random allocation, randomized or randomly assigned)
Introduction Background	Scientific background and explanation of rationale
Methods Participants	Eligibility criteria for participants and the settings and locations where the data were collected
Interventions	Precise details of the interventions intended for each group and how and when they were actually administered
Objectives	Specific objectives and hypotheses
Outcomes	Clearly defined primary and secondary outcome measures and, when applicable, any methods used to enhance the quality of measurements (e.g. multiple observations, training of assessors)
Sample size	How sample size was determined and, when applicable, explanation of any interim analyses and stopping rules
Randomization – sequence generation	Method used to generate the random allocation sequence, including details of any restrictions (e.g. blocking, stratification)
Randomization – allocation concealment	Method used to implement the random allocation sequence (e.g. numbered containers or central telephone), clarifying whether or not the sequence was concealed until interventions were assigned
Randomization – implementation	Who generated the allocation sequence, who enrolled participants and who assigned participants to their groups
Blinding (masking)	Whether or not participants, those administering the interventions and those assessing the outcomes were blinded to group assignment When relevant, how the success of blinding was evaluated
Statistical methods	Statistical methods used to compare groups for primary outcome(s); methods for additional analyses, such as subgroup analyses and adjusted analyses
Results Participant flow	Flow of participants through each stage (a diagram is strongly recommended). Specifically, for each group report the numbers of participants randomly assigned, receiving intended treatment, completing the study protocol and analysed for the primary outcome Describe protocol deviations from study as planned, together with reasons
Recruitment	Dates defining the periods of recruitment and follow-up
Baseline data	Baseline demographic and clinical characteristics of each group
Numbers analysed	Number of participants (denominator) in each group included in each analysis and whether the analysis was by intention-to-treat. State the results in absolute numbers when feasible (e.g. 10/20, not 50%)
Outcomes and estimation	For each primary and secondary outcome, a summary of results for each group, and the estimated effect size and its precision (e.g. 95% confidence interval)

Table 9.3　*(cont.)*

Paper section and topic	Description
Ancillary analyses	Address multiplicity by reporting any other analyses performed, including subgroup analyses and adjusted analyses, indicating those pre-specified and those exploratory
Adverse events	All important adverse events or side effects in each intervention group
Discussion Interpretation	Interpretation of the results, taking into account study hypotheses, sources of potential bias or imprecision and the dangers associated with multiplicity of analyses and outcomes
Generalizability	Generalizability (external validity) of the trial findings
Overall evidence	General interpretation of the results in the context of current evidence

*The CONSORT statement is an important research tool that takes an evidence-based approach to improve the quality of reports of randomized trials. It is published on the internet and can be found at http://www.consort-statement.org/.

16. Ethical considerations are paramount. Harmful interventions, withholding a recognised beneficial treatment and prolonging a trial when the outcome is unlikely to change must be avoided.

9.9　References

Holmes MA, Cockcroft PD, Booth CE, Heath MF (2005) Controlled clinical trial of the effect of a homoeopathic nosode on the somatic cell counts in the milk of clinically normal dairy cows. *Vet. Rec.* Apr 30 **156**(18): 565–7.

Kimmel SE, Michel KE, Hess RS, Ward CR (2000) Effects of insoluble and soluble dietary fiber on glycemic control in dogs with naturally occurring insulin-dependent diabetes mellitus. *J. Am. Vet. Med. Assoc.* **216**(7): 1076–81.

Lockwood PW, Johnson JC, Katz TL (2003) Clinical efficacy of flunixin, carprofen and ketoprofen as adjuncts to the antibacterial treatment of bovine respiratory disease. *Vet. Rec.* **152**(13): 392–4.

Noordhuizen JPTM, Frankena K, Ploeger H, Nell T (1993) (eds) Field trial and error. *Proceedings of the International Seminar with Workshops on the Design, Conduct and Interpretation of Field Trials*, Berg en Dal, Netherlands, 27–28 April 1993, Epidecon, Wageningen.

Olivry T, Rivrerre C, Jackson HA, Murphy KM, Davidson G, Sousa CA (2002) Cyclosporine decreases skin lesions and pruritus in dogs with alopic dermatitis; a blinded randomized prednisolone-controlled trial. *Vet Dermatol* **13**(2): 77–87.

Thrusfield M (2005) Clinical trials. In: *Veterinary Epidemiology*, 3rd edn, Blackwell Publishing, Oxford, p 292.

Whittem TL, Johnson AL, Smith CW, Schaeffer DJ, Coolman BR, Averill SM, Cooper TK, Merkin GR (1999) Effect of perioperative prophylactic antimicrobial treatment in dogs undergoing elective orthopedic surgery. *J. Am. Vet. Med. Assoc.* **215**(2): 212–16.

Woodward M (2005) Intervention studies. In: *Epidemiology: Study and Data Analysis*, Chapman and Hall/CRC, London, P 339–41.

9.10　Further reading

Ajetunmobi O (2002) Critical appraisal of randomised clinical trials. In: *Making Sense of Critical Appraisal*, Arnold, London, pp 122–45.

Dahoo IR, Waltner-Toews D (1985) Interpreting Clinical Research: Part I. General Considerations. *Compendium of Continuing Education* **7** (9): S474–S477.

Dahoo IR, Waltner-Toews D (1985) Interpreting Clinical Research: Part II. Descriptive and Experimental Studies. *Compendium of Continuing Education* **7** (9): S513–S519.

Dahoo IR, Waltner-Toews D (1985) Interpreting Clinical Research: Part 3 Observational Studies and Interpretation of Results. *Compendium of Continuing Education* **7** (9): S605–S613.

Fletcher RH, Fletcher SW, Wagner EH (1996) Treatment. In: *Clinical Epidemiology (The Essentials)*,

3rd edn, Williams and Wilkins, Baltimore, pp 136–64.

Friedman LM, Furberg CD, DeMets DL (1998) *Fundamentals of Clinical Trials*, Springer, New York.

Hulley SB, Cummings SR, Browner WS, Grady DG, Newman TB (2007) Designing a randomised trial. In: *Designing Clinical Research*, 3rd edn, Lippincott Williams and Wilkins, Philadelphia, pp 127–146.

Hulley SB, Newman TB, Cummings SR (2001) Designing an experiment: clinical trials II. In: *Designing Clinical Research*, 2nd edn, Lippincott Williams and Wilkins, Philadelphia, pp 157–74.

Lund EM, James MJ, Neaton JD (1994) Clinical trial design: veterinary perspectives. *J. Vet. Int. Med.* **5**: 317–22.

Lund EM, James MJ, Neaton JD (1998) Veterinary randomized clinical trial reporting: a review of the small animals literature. *J. Vet. Intern. Med.* **12**: 57–60.

Medical Research Council (1998) Guidelines for good clinical practice in clinical trials, Medical Research Council (includes the Helsinki declaration). MRC website.

Munz M, Cox A (2001) Conducting clinical trials in practice. *In Practice* **9**: 551–3.

Pollock SJ (2004) *Clinical Trials: A Practical Approach*, John Wiley and Sons Ltd, Chichester.

Sanderson MW (2006) Designing and Running Clinical Trials of Farms in Barnyard Epidemiology and Performance Assessment, Reugg P L (ed), *Veterinary Clinics North America* **22**(1): 103–24.

Smith RD (2006) Design and evaluation. In: *Veterinary Clinical Epidemiology*, 3rd edn, CRC Press, London, pp 127–35.

Thrusfield M (2005) Clinical trials. In: *Veterinary Epidemiology*, 3rd edn, Blackwell Publishing, Oxford, pp 2289–304.

Woodward M (2005) Intervention studies. In: *Epidemiology: Study and Data Analysis*, Chapman and Hall/CRC, London, pp 335–80.

9.11 MCQs

1 **An important feature of a randomized controlled trial is:**

(a) it is expensive
(b) there are at least two groups, one of which is a treatment group and one a control group
(c) it can be published
(d) subjects are readily available
(e) it is easy to perform.

2 **Which of the following is a disadvantage of a randomized controlled clinical trial?**

(a) Random allocation reduces the risk of bias and is the most powerful method of eliminating known and unknown confounding variables.
(b) The allocation of subjects and the number of subjects allocated to each treatment is planned.
(c) Cause precedes effect.
(d) It is the most powerful study design for data collection.
(e) Sometimes it is unethical to allow for an untreated control group due to the severity of the effects of withholding an effective treatment.

3 **Which of the following is an advantage of the cross-over design?**

(a) The number of animals can usually be reduced compared to a randomized controlled trial.
(b) Treatments with persistent actions confound the results.
(c) It is suitable only for long-term conditions for which treatment provides only short-term relief, e.g. chronic arthritis.
(d) Statistical appraisal is simple.
(e) It has greater validity than parallel randomized controlled trials.

4 **Sample size calculations are important because:**

(a) they indicate the minimum number of participants required to achieve a specified power
(b) they indicate the number of participants required to achieve a representative sample of a target population
(c) they indicate the maximum samples that can be recruited for the study budget
(d) all the above
(e) none of the above.

5 **An important criterion for exclusion would be:**

(a) prior knowledge that a treatment may be unsafe or have an adverse side effect in a defined subset of the target population

(b) prior knowledge that allocation to the placebo group would adversely affect the progression of a disease

(c) subjects in whom the treatment is unlikely to have any beneficial effect

(d) subjects who are unlikely to comply with the treatment, recording of measurements or be available for follow-up

(e) all of the above.

6 Randomization of participants in a trial ensures that:

(a) patients are allocated to each intervention without selection bias

(b) the investigator does not know the allocation of subjects to treatments

(c) owners do not know which treatment their pet will receive

(d) confounding variables are unevenly distributed between treatment groups

(e) investigators are randomly allocated to treatment groups.

7 Double blinding ensures that:

(a) the investigator does not know the treatment a trial participant is receiving

(b) the owner does not know the treatment a trial participant is receiving

(c) the investigator and the owner do not know the treatment a trial participant is receiving

(d) all the above

(e) none of the above.

8 Superiority trials are:

(a) trials that have a better design

(b) trials that have larger sample sizes

(c) trials that are designed to investigate if a treatment is superior to another treatment

(d) trials that are performed in a controlled environment

(e) samples that are more representative of the target population.

9 Which of the following treatment factors are important to consider when designing a clinical trial?

(a) Effectiveness and safety of the drug.

(b) Feasibility of blinding.

(c) Whether different dose rates will be studied.

(d) Sample population and the generalizability of the results.

(e) All of the above.

10 Which of the following would not increase compliance?

(a) Detailed treatment instructions.

(b) Financial inducements.

(c) Motivational meetings.

(d) A long study period and a complex treatment regimen.

(e) A short study period and a simple treatment regimen.

9.12   MCQ answers

1. (b); 2. (e); 3. (a); 4. (a); 5. (e); 6. (a); 7. (c); 8. (c); 9. (e); 10 (d)

10

STUDIES ON DIAGNOSTIC TESTS

119

Objectives

After reading this chapter readers should:

- understand the utility of diagnostic tests (sensitivity and specificity)
- understand clinically relevant questions that can be asked about a test
- be able to plan and implement a study on a diagnostic test.

10.1   Introduction

Diagnostic tests may take the form of clinical examinations, microbiological isolations, serological tests, pathophysiological assessment, gross and histopathology, and ultrasonic and radiographic interpretation. They are an important component of the diagnostic process. They may be used to estimate the probability of disease, indicate the value of a risk factor and provide information regarding the prognosis of a patient. Descriptive statistics such as sensitivity, specificity and confidence interval are crucial in defining the clinical worth of a test result. Most designs to evaluate clinical tests are descriptive and observational. Case-control and cross-sectional designs are usually used.

Statistical differences between the target disease group and the comparative group may not be clinically useful and may be clinically difficult to interpret. Studies that estimate the precision, the performance (sensitivity, specificity), feasibility, likelihood ratios, predictive values, cost-benefit and risks in performing the test are more useful in evaluating the clinical significance and performance of the test. Consistent results are important to enable interpretations to be accurately standardized. The information must be useful in shaping treatments by predicting clinical outcomes by increasing the likelihood of a correct diagnosis or by being cheaper and safer than an existing test.

There are many different (and possibly confusing) ways in which the performance of a test may be reported (Fig. 10.1). The test attempts to identify two populations: the animals free of the disease and the animals with the disease. Measures of performance look at four different possibilities:

(a)   The test can be positive in animals with the disease (a true positive result).

(b)   The test can be positive in animals free of the disease (a false positive).

(c)   The test can be negative in animals with the disease (a false negative).

(d)   The test can be negative in animals free of the disease (a true negative).

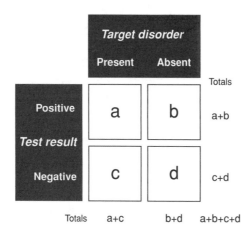

$$\text{SPECIFICITY} = \frac{a}{a + c}$$

$$\text{SENSITIVITY} = \frac{d}{b + d}$$

The likelihood ratio for a positive test result

$$\text{LR+} = \frac{\text{sensitivity}}{1 - \text{specificity}}$$

The likelihood ratio for a negative test result

$$\text{LR-} = \frac{1 - \text{sensitivity}}{\text{specificity}}$$

Figure 10.1 A contingency table showing how the results of a diagnostic test using a case-control study design can be analysed.

Ideally we want to maximize the instances of (a) and (d), while minimizing the instances of (b) and (c).

Sensitivity is the proportion of diseased animals with a positive result.

Specificity is the proportion of animals without the disease with a negative result.

We combine these measures into the indicators of the overall efficiency of a test by calculating likelihood ratio. Likelihood ratios enable us to convert a pre-test probability of disease to a post-test probability.

The positive likelihood ratio is the ratio of the proportion of positive-test animals who have the disease (sensitivity) to the proportion of positive-test animals who do not have the disease (1 – specificity). The negative likelihood ratio similarly gives us the ratio of false negatives (1 – sensitivity) to true negatives (specificity).

It is important to realize that the sensitivity and specificity (and thus likelihood ratios) are absolute measures of a test's performance; however, the post-test probability is determined by the amount of disease present in the population in the first place, the pre-test probability. The pre-test probability is numerically the same as the prevalence of the disease (conceptually pre-test probability applies to an individual, whereas prevalence applies to a population).

From all this, it is clear that we need to know how well the test performs (i.e. sensitivity and specificity) and prevalence data in order to answer the two important questions: what does a positive result mean for our patient and what does a negative result mean for our patient?

A test is a variable that can be measured. Test results may be nominal (positive or negative), ordinal (weak, intermediate, strong) or interval (serum titre). Clinical signs, biochemical parameters and antibody titres are all examples of test results. It is advisable to record ordinal or continuous measures if possible to capture the information in detail even if these

are reduced to categorical measures during the analysis.

Accuracy is the proportion of all tests both positive and negative that are correct for a defined population of test animals. This accuracy for the population of test animals may or may not represent the accuracy of the test in the target population. In case-control studies the accuracy of the tests will not be transferable to the target population although the values of the sensitivity and specificity will be. In cross-sectional studies, where the disease prevalence in the target population will be mirrored by the sample, the accuracy estimate for the test population will apply to the target population. Precision is also an important consideration but it is rarely reported. Precision is the agreement between the results when the tests are repeated on the same samples.

10.2 Measuring the specificity, sensitivity and prevalence

In order to establish the importance of the result we need to have values for the sensitivity and specificity. Test results are required for two groups of animals: animals with the target disease and animals without the disease. The presence or absence of disease in all the participants should be defined by a gold standard test that is independent of the test undergoing evaluation.

Ideally a gold standard is a test which has specificity and sensitivity of 100%. It enables animals to be categorized absolutely. In reality it is the best test we can use given the study limitations. It may be histopathology, gross pathology, microbiological culture, virus isolation, polymerase chain reaction or the opinion of an expert.

In many cases the sensitivity and specificity are measured using a case-control design and the prevalence is measured using a cross-sectional study. Cross-sectional studies can be used to derive the sensitivity, specificity and prevalence. Sample size is important. Confidence intervals can be defined for a proportion. Assessments should be made to ensure that for a given sensitivity enough participants have been used to define sensible confidence intervals. The investigators should be blinded when performing the test under investigation and the gold standard.

It is important to note that the sensitivity of a test can vary depending on the clinical stage of disease in the animals. For example in the ELISA test for *Mycobacterium paratuberculosis* in cattle, as the clinical severity of the disease increases so does the sensitivity of the test. Specificity is defined as the proportion of animals without the disease giving a negative test result. This is often defined with regard to healthy participants or non-diseased participants. This may be valid for screening tests but not for diagnostic tests. The specificity has to be defined for the subpopulation that does not have the target disease. This should include animals with other diseases in the target population. There is a danger when performing case-control studies, in order to define sensitivities and specificities, that these clinical profile criteria for participants will not be observed. It is easier and simpler to define two categories of patient (diseased and healthy) and neglect their appropriate clinical profiles. Cross-sectional studies are therefore preferable as they automatically select animals with appropriate disease profiles defined by the inclusion and exclusion criteria. The disadvantage is that for rare diseases a large sample has to be taken to get a large enough diseased sample size.

The participants in the study must include individuals with all the clinically important forms of the disease or stages of disease in the target population that will be presented for testing. They should also be represented in the same proportions as the target population. If these conditions are met then the measured sensitivity will be independent of the prevalence of the target disease. The participants that do not have the disease must also have the same range, prevalence and proportions of other diseases, and clinical stage presentations as the animals in the target populations that will be presented for testing.

Provided the relative proportions of the non-target diseases of the participants are representative of the target population, the specificity is independent of the absolute prevalence of the non-target diseases.

10.2.1   Case-control design to measure sensitivity and specificity

The case-control study design is described in Chapter 8. This design cannot measure prevalence. The result can be analysed using a contingency table and the formulae for sensitivity and specificity and the liklihood ratios for a negative and positive test results are shown in Fig. 10.1.

Defining the sensitivity and specificity will provide the clinician with the change in odds given a test result (i.e. the likelihood ratio for a positive test and the likelihood ratio for a negative test), but without an estimate of the disease prevalence the probability of the animal having or not having the disease given a test (positive and negative predictive values) cannot be computed. An estimate of the prevalence is sometimes available from other sources. Accuracy can be defined but is only applicable to the test population sample of animals that are not representative of the prevalence of disease in the target testing population.

10.2.2   Cross-sectional study design to measure specificity, sensitivity and prevalence

The prevalence, specificity and sensitivity may be measured at the same time by performing a cross-sectional study. The cross-section study design is described in Chapter 8. From this information the clinician can answer the questions: what does a positive result mean for our patient and what does a negative result mean for our patient? A contingency table showing how the result of a cross-section study of a diagnostic test can be analysed is shown in Fig. 10.2.

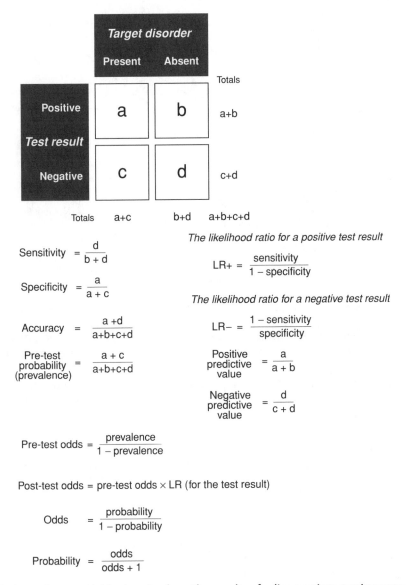

Figure 10.2 A contingency table showing how the results of a diagnostic test using a cross-sectional study design can be analysed.

10.3 Tests with continuous measures

Many tests have a result that is a continuous value, for example biochemical measures and ELISA tests. In these circumstances a cut-off value can be chosen below which the test is deemed to be negative and above which the test is deemed to be positive. The sensitivity and specificity of each cut-off value can be determined, giving a series of values defined by the cut-off value. The sensitivity and specificity values obtained for a range of cut-off points can be presented graphically on a receiver–operator curve (ROC). The

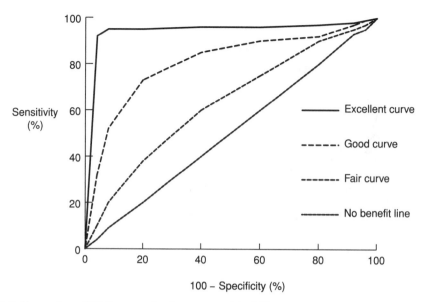

Figure 10.3 Examples of ROC curves for four tests with different accuracies.

horizontal axis is (1 – specificity) and the vertical axis is the sensitivity. The total area under the ROC represents the probability of the test correctly identifying true positives and true negatives, i.e. the test accuracy. The test with the greatest area under the curve is the most accurate. The point on the ROC nearest to the point on the y-axis that represents a specificity of 100% (1.0) and sensitivity of 100% (1.0) is the cut-off value that will give the greatest accuracy. This is illustrated in Figs 10.3 and 10.4. This cut-off point is more readily appreciated using a two-graph receiver–operator curve analysis (TG-ROC) this illustrated in Figs 10.5 and 10.6. The cut-off point with the greatest accuracy is given by the intersection of the sensitivity and specificity in Fig. 10.6. This cut-off point results in the least number of diagnostic errors.

Figure 10.4 shows ROC plots for four serum enzymes, alanine transferase, alanine transferase P5P apoenzyme, aspartate aminotranferase and aspartate aminotranferase P5P apoenzyme, and the hemolytic index for 37 diseased dogs (liver or muscle disease) and 155 clinically normal dogs (Gardner and Greiner, 2006) using data from Stokol and Erb (1998).

The area under the curve (AUC) is a measure of the accuracy and ranges between 0.5 and 1.0. A perfect test has a score of 1.0 and a test which provides no additional information has a score of 0.5. An arbitrary interpretation of the AUC value which may be useful clinically is: low $0.5 < AUC \leq 0.7$, moderate $0.7 < AUC \leq 0.9$ or high $0.9 < AUC \leq 1.0$ (Swets, 1988). ROC curves also enable tests with different scales of measure to be compared, as shown in Table 10.1.

Table 10.1 Area under the curve (AUC) and 95% confidence interval (CI) for four serum enzymes (ALT, alanine transferase; ALTP5P, alanine transferase P5P apoenzyme; AST aspartate aminotranferase; ASTP5P, aspartate aminotranferase P5P apoenzyme) and the hemolytic index for 37 diseased dogs (liver or muscle disease) and 155 clinically normal dogs. (Gardner and Greiner, 2006) using data from Stokel and Erb (1998).

Serum enzyme or index	AUC	95% CI
ALT	0.935	0.883–0.968
ALTP5P	0.943	0.893–0.974
AST	0.912	0.856–0.952
ASTP5P	0.908	0.850–0.949
Haemolytic index	0.500	0.418–0.582

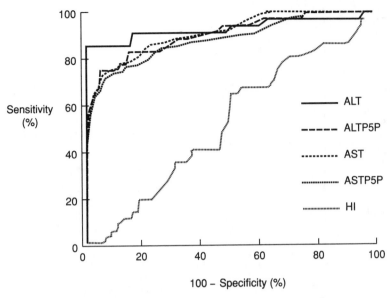

Figure 10.4 ROC plots for four serum enzymes (ALT, alanine transferase; ALTP5P, alanine transferase P5P apoenzyme; AST, aspartate aminotranferase; ASTP5P, aspartate aminotranferase P5P apoenzyme) and the hemolytic index (HI) for 37 diseased dogs (liver or muscle disease) and 155 clinically normal dogs (Gardner and Greiner, 2006) using data from Stokol and Erb (1998).

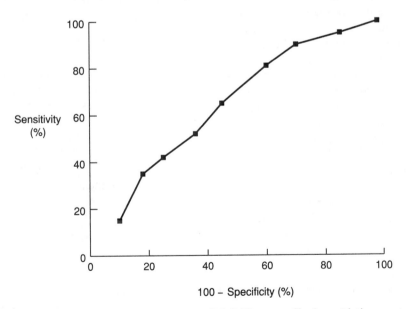

Figure 10.5 Example of a receiver–operator curve (ROC). The cut-off value with the greatest accuracy is difficult to identify.

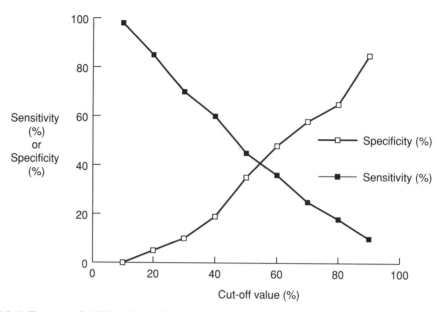

Figure 10.6 Two-graph ROC analysis. The intersection of the sensitivity and specificity lines indicate the cut-off value with the greatest accuracy.

In clinical medicine the greatest accuracy or the test with the least diagnostic error may not have the cut-off value that is the most useful. It is also important to remember that the accuracy is dependent on the prevalence of the disease (pre-test odds). The relative costs (impact) of false positive and false negative results are often very different. For example, with BSE detection in cattle we want a test with a high sensitivity to ensure we do not miss any cases and we are prepared to accept that some false positive results will occur. If we are contemplating using an invasive technique with a high risk to the patient, we may wish to be very certain that the patient has the condition, so a cut-off point with a high degree of specificity may be used. This reflects the SpPin and SnNout mnemonic:

- For a test with a high specificity (Sp), if the test is positive then it rules the diagnosis in.
- For a test with a high sensitivity (Sn), if the test is negative it rules out the condition.

10.4   Studies that compare two tests to find out which is better

The gold standard test can be expensive or invasive. A cheaper design to discover which of two or more tests is the most accurate but avoids having to use the gold standard test on all patients is called tandem testing. Both tests are done on a random sample of patients who may or may not have the disease. The gold standard is then applied to the patients who test positive on either test. This does not yield the sensitivity or the specificity of the test.

10.5   Prognostic tests

Prognostic tests are performed on patients that already have the disease. The outcome is what happens to them in terms of longevity or the progression of the clinical disease. Prospective or retrospective cohort designs can be used. In prospective studies the test is done at the start of the study and the subjects are followed over time and monitored for the outcome of interest. Observer blinding is important in prospective studies to avoid bias. In retrospective studies stored samples are used for the test under evaluation. The subjects who develop the disease of interest are known at the start of the study. The nested case-control design is a useful design if the outcome of interest is rare and the test expensive.

The analysis of prognostic tests for disease is similar to that used for other cohort studies. Relative risk or absolute risk can be used for set time period follow-ups. Survival analysis is more appropriate if mortality is the outcome measure over time.

10.6 Studies of test reproducibility (precision)

Reproducibility is the same as precision. There can be high precision but poor accuracy. For example, two observers may have good agreement but they may both be wrong. Studies of precision do not require a gold standard.

Intra-observer variability describes the differences in the results obtained when a laboratory or observer performs a test on the same sample (patient) at different times, for example the same radiograph may be examined twice by the same observer with a 1-week interval between examinations. Inter-observer variability describes the differences in the results obtained when two different observers examine the same sample, for example a radiograph. If intra- or inter-observer reproducibility is poor, it is unlikely that the test will be useful unless automated methods of measuring are devised or appropriate training is provided.

For tests that use samples that may have undergone different processing methods, such as for histopathology, a study may investigate the changes in the agreement depending on which method of processing was used. It is important that tests that rely on varying methodologies are described in detail when the study is submitted for publication.

Cross-sectional studies can be used to compare the test results from more than one observer. The simplest statistical measure of inter-observer agreement with categorical data is the concordance rate. The concordance rate is the proportion of observations on which the observers agree. This statistic, however, does not account for agreement by chance and a better measure of inter-observer agreement is the kappa statistic. This measures the extent of the agreement once chance has been taken into account. Kappa values range from −1 (perfect disagreement) to +1 (perfect agreement); 0 indicates the result was exactly as expected by chance.

Descriptive statistics of inter-observer variability using continuous variable measures with paired measurements may include the mean differences between paired measurements and the distribution of the measurement standard error. Comparison of multiple observers or laboratory machines can be summarized using the coefficient of variation.

10.7 Studies on the impact of a test on patient outcomes

Does testing make a difference to the patient and/or owner? Diagnostic yield studies are studies that investigate the impact of using tests on the clinical outcomes of patients. This may be as a result of early treatment or changes in treatment that follow on from a test result.

Before and after studies investigate the impact on clinical decision making once the result of the test is known. Changes in the clinical management may not be of benefit to the patient and these will have to be measured if the study is to answer that additional question. These studies can also yield the effort:yield ratio. This

Table 10.2 Questions to determine the usefulness of a clinical test, possible designs to answer them and statistics for reporting the results.

Research question	Study design	Descriptive statistic

How reproducible are the test results?	Intra-observer variability
	Inter-observer variability
	Intra-laboratory variability
	Inter-laboratory variability
		Proportion agreement
		Kappa
		Coefficient
		  of variation
		Mean and distribution of
		  differences

Is the test accurate?	Cross-sectional study Case-control study Cohort study (test result vs gold standard)	Sensitivity Specificity Predictive values Likelihood ratio ROC curve

What is the clinical relevance of a test?	Diagnostic yield study
	Comparison of clinical
	  decision-making pre- and
	  post-test results
		Proportion of abnormal or
		  discordant results
		Proportion of tests that lead to a
		  decision change

What are the costs, risks and acceptability of the test?	Prospective study Retrospective studies	Average cost Number of adverse effects Client compliance rate

What are the clinical outcomes resulting from the test?	Randomized controlled studies
	Cohort study
	Case-control study (predictor
	  variable is receiving the test,
	  outcome variable is morbidity,
	  mortality, cost, etc.)
		Risk ratio
		Odds ratio
		Hazard ratio
		Number needed to treat
		Number needed to harm

involves measuring the beneficial outcomes of performing the test and also measuring the effort needed to obtain these beneficial outcomes. The value of the test can then be appraised. Examples of low yield and benefit may be testing the foremilk of every quarter of every cow at every milking to check for visible signs of mastitis. In most herds the number of additional mastitis cases detected by this method is very low. These studies are often used with screening tests to indicate the likely benefit.

10.8 Studies on the feasibility, costs and additional risks of tests

Studies on the feasibility, costs and risks of tests are important if implementation in clinical practice is proposed or if a national testing programme is contemplated. These studies are usually descriptive and are summarized using simple statistics such as means, standard deviations, medians, ranges and frequency distributions.

10.9 Summary of clinical test study designs

Table 10.2 indicates the range of clinical questions that determine the usefulness of a test, the designs that can be used to provide meaningful answers and the statistical measures for reporting the results.

10.10 Sources of bias in the evaluation of diagnostic tests

10.10.1 The gold standard

The gold standard is rarely absolute and therefore the sensitivity and specificity values generated are relative to the standard test used rather than absolute. Bias is therefore introduced.

10.10.2 Inadequate sample size

Tables indicating the 95% confidence intervals for a given proportion using different sample sizes are useful when deciding on the sample size required. Pilot studies may also be a useful predictor of appropriate sample sizes.

10.10.3 Inappropriate exclusion

Great care is needed not to bias the results when a result is not obtained or the result is indeterminate. Criteria for exclusion need to be considered very carefully and made explicit in the protocols and reports.

10.10.4 Generalizability of the results

It is important that the reporting of the study is sufficiently detailed to reflect potential differences that may occur if the test is used elsewhere. Inter-observer studies are important safeguards for this potential error.

10.10.5 Spectrum bias

The diseased category of participants should reflect the severity profiles and proportions present in the target population. Alternatively, sensitivities and specificities can be defined by clinical stage, in which case the group of diseased participants should be at the same stage as defined by a detailed case descriptor.

The non-diseased category should contain healthy individuals if a screening test is being evaluated. If a diagnostic test is being evaluated then the study should report the proportions and clinical profiles of other diseases and healthy animals present in the target populations. The target population can be defined by the investigator giving the criteria to which the test results apply. Care is needed not to define a population to which the results will never apply in clinical

practice. It is important to avoid samples that indicate extremes, such as comparing the performance of a test in severe categories of the disease against healthy patients.

10.10.6 Investigator bias

There must be consistency in the application of the gold standard to ensure there is no bias in the classification of the participants. This is especially true when a post-test result post-mortem is used as a gold standard or radiographic analysis. To avoid this bias the results of the test must not be revealed to the pathologist undertaking the post-mortem or the observer performing the subjective interpretation. It is crucial that in tests involving subjective judgement the tester is blinded to the category to which the patient belongs. It is also important that the observer is not privy to additional patient information that may increase the probability of the observer deducing the likely disease status of the patient.

If the investigator knows the categories of the participants and the test involves a clinical measurement then observer bias is possible. Blinding may be possible but if the diseased group demonstrates clinical signs of disease compared to the control group then the use of two blinded operators is preferable.

10.10.7 Subjective tests

Some tests involve subjective interpretation, such as the examination of radiographs for a specific lesion or the examination of an animal for diagnostic clinical signs. Inter-observer variation will result in different specificities and sensitivities for the test, depending on the tester. Intra-observer agreement may be poor if the subjective interpretation is inconsistent.

10.10.8 Complex laboratory tests

Some tests involve long and complex methods that require a high level of technical skill to perform. The competence and training of technical staff can influence the validity of the test. Studies may be needed to estimate the degree of systematic error in some tests which fall into this category in order to estimate the criteria required to implement the tests.

10.11   Checklist for studies of diagnostic tests (modified from Fletcher et al., 1996)

1. Have definitions of a positive test result and a negative test result been decided on and documented? If continuous measures are to be used, cut-off points and ROC should be used during the analysis.
2. What is the gold standard to be used to establish the presence or absence of the target disease in all participants?
3. Does the clinical profile or spectrum of patients represent the target testing population in both groups (target disease, others)?
4. Will there be an unbiased assessment of test and disease status? Bias can occur if the test result is determined with knowledge of the disease status and vice versa.
5. Will the experimental design be able to measure the specificity and the sensitivity of the test?
6. What scale of measure will be used: categorical, ordinal or continuous?
7. Will the experimental design be able to determine the prevalence of the target disease (cross-sectional studies) so that predictive values can be presented?

10.12   Examples

The following abstracts of published scientific papers are of studies evaluating tests. They indicate the applications of some of the principles described in this section.

Six criteria for rabies diagnosis in living dogs (Tepsumethanon et al., 2005)

Objective: The authors studied the predictive value of six criteria for clinical diagnosis of rabies in living dogs. *Design*: Identify and test the criteria

in a retrospective and prospective study. *Material and method*: Both studies were conducted at the Rabies Diagnostic Unit, Queen Saovabha Memorial Institute, Thai Red Cross Society, Bangkok. The authors reviewed 1,170 dogs that were kept under observation for 10 days after they exhibited abnormal behavior. To test the predictive value of the six criteria, a prospective study involving 450 rabies suspected dogs was also performed. *Results and conclusion*: The six criteria demonstrated 90.2% sensitivity, 96.2% specificity and 94.6% accuracy for the clinical diagnosis of rabies. They can be used for a presumptive diagnosis and may help in prioritizing post-exposure treatments and institute urgent rabies control measures.

Diagnostic value of fasting plasma ammonia and bile acid concentrations in the identification of portosystemic shunting in dogs (Gerritzen-Bruning et al., 2006)

Portosystemic shunting occurs frequently either as congenital anomalies of the portal vein (PVA) or as acquired shunting (AS) due to portal hypertension secondary to parenchymal liver disease or portal vein thrombosis. The 2 most commonly used screening tests for portosystemic shunting are bile acid and plasma ammonia concentrations. The purpose of this study was to compare the 12-hour fasting plasma ammonia (AMM) and bile acid concentration (BA) as tests for diagnosing portosystemic shunting. Medical records of 337 dogs were used in which AMM and BA were measured simultaneously and in which portosystemic shunting was confirmed or excluded. These dogs were divided into 2 groups (group 1: portosystemic shunting present, n = 153, and group 2: portosystemic shunting absent, n = 184). Group 1 was subdivided into 2 subgroups (group 1a: PVA, n = 132 and group 1b: AS, n = 21). The sensitivity of AMM in detecting PVA was 100% and of BA was 92.2%. For portosystemic shunting in general (PVA or AS), the sensitivity of AMM was 98% and that of BA was 88.9%. The specificity in the total population of AMM was 89.1% and that of BA was 67.9%. If only dogs with liver diseases were included with (n = 153) or without (n = 28) shunting, the specificity of AMM to detect shunting was 89.3% and that of BA was 17.9%. In conclusion, AMM is a highly sensitive and specific parameter to detect PVA and portosystemic shunting in a general population and in dogs with liver disease, whereas BA is somewhat less sensitive and considerably less specific.

Development and Bayesian evaluation of an ELISA to detect specific antibodies to *Sarcoptes scabiei* var suis in the meat juice of pigs (Vercruysse et al., 2006)

Samples of ear scrapings, serum and diaphragmatic muscle were collected from 271 fattening pigs at the slaughterhouse. The scrapings were examined for the presence of mites, and tests for specific antibodies to *Sarcoptes scabiei* var suis in the serum and meat juice were made with an experimental ELISA. The cut-off value for the meat-juice ELISA was estimated at an optical density of 0.5 by receiver operating characteristic curve analysis, on the basis of the cut-off value for the serum ELISA of 0.4. The results of the three tests were used in a Bayesian model to estimate the characteristics of each test. The specificity of the tests of the ear scrapings was considered to be 1 and their sensitivity was estimated by Bayesian analysis to be 0.86, with a 95 per cent confidence interval (CI) of 0.73 to 0.99. The sensitivity of the meat juice ELISA (0.71, 95 per cent CI 0.6 to 0.8) and its specificity (0.77, 95 per cent CI 0.66 to 0.89) were comparable with the sensitivity (0.73, 95 per cent CI 0.6 to 0.8) and specificity (0.81, 95 per cent CI 0.69 to 0.95) of the serum ELISA.

Prognostic value of clinicopathologic variables obtained at admission and effect of antiendotoxin plasma on survival in septic and critically ill foals (Peek et al., 2006)

This prospective study compared survival rates of critically ill and septic foals receiving 1 of 2 different types of commercial equine plasma and analyzed admission variables as possible predictors of survival. Standardized clinical, hema-tologic, biochemical, and hemostatic admission data were collected and foals received either conventional commercially available hyperimmune equine plasma or equine plasma specifically rich in antiendotoxin antibodies in a double-blinded, coded fashion. Sepsis was defined as true bacteremia or sepsis score >11. Overall survival rate to discharge was 72% (49/68). Foals that were nonbacteremic and demonstrated a sepsis score of < or = 11 at admission had a 95% (18/19) survival rate. The survival rate to discharge for septic foals was 28/49 (57%), with truly bacteremic foals having a survival rate of 58% (14/24), whereas that for nonbacteremic, septic foals was 56% (14/25). Sensitivity and specificity for sepsis score >11 as a predictor of bacteremia were 74 and 52%, respectively. For the entire study population, a higher survival rate to discharge was documented for those foals receiving hyperimmune plasma rich in antiendotoxin antibodies (P = .012, odds ratio [OR] 6.763, 95% confidence interval [CI]: 1.311, 34.903). Administration of plasma rich in antiendotoxin antibodies also was associated with greater survival in septic foals (P = .019, OR 6.267, 95% CI: 1.186, 33.109). Statistical analyses demonstrated that, among 53 clinical and clinicopathologic admission variables, high sepsis score (P < .001), low measured IgG concentration (P = .01), high fibrinogen concentration (P = .018), low segmented neutrophil count (P = .028), and low total red blood cell numbers (P = .048) were the most significant predictors of overall mortality.

Accuracy of increased thyroid activity during pertechnetate scintigraphy by subcutaneous injection for diagnosing hyperthyroidism in cats (Page et al., 2006)

Our purpose was to determine the accuracy of increased thyroid activity for diagnosing hyperthyroidism in cats suspected of having that disease during pertechnetate scintigraphy using subcutaneous rather than intravenous radioisotope administration. Increased thyroid activity was determined by two methods: the thyroid:salivary ratio (T:S) and visual inspection.

These assessments were made on the ventral scintigram of the head and neck. Scintigraphy was performed by injecting sodium pertechnetate (111 MBq, SQ) in the right-dorsal-lumbar region; static-acquisition images were obtained 20 min after injection. We used 49 cats; 34 (69%) had hyperthyroidism based on serum-chemistry analysis. Using a Wilcoxon's rank-sum test, a significant difference ($P < 0.0001$) was detected in the T:S between cats with and without hyperthyroidism. Using a decision criterion of 2.0 for the T:S, the test accurately predicted hyperthyroidism in 32/34 cats (sensitivity, 94%; 95% confidence interval (CI), 85–100%) and correctly predicted that hyperthyroidism was absent in 15/15 cats (specificity, 100%; CI, 97–100%). Using visual inspection, the test accurately predicted hyperthyroidism in 34/34 cats (sensitivity, 100%; CI, 99–100%) and correctly predicted that hyperthyroidism was absent in 12/15 cats (specificity, 80%; CI, 56–100%). The positive and negative predictive values were high for a wide range of prevalence of hyperthyroidism. And, the test had excellent agreement within and between examiners. Therefore, detecting increased thyroid activity during pertechnetate scintigraphy by subcutaneous injection is an accurate and reproducible test for feline hyperthyroidism.

Comparison and standardisation of serological methods for the diagnosis of *Neospora caninum* infection in bovines (von Blumroder et al., 2004)

Various existing serological tests were compared with a standard panel of 523 sera in a multicentred study across Europe. Well characterised sera from animals that were experimentally or naturally infected with *Neospora caninum* as well as sera from cattle deemed uninfected with *N. caninum* were provided by the participants of the study and analysed in several commercial (CHEKIT Dr. Bommeli/Intervet, CIVTEST BOVIS NEOSPORA Hipra, Cypress Diagnostics C.V., Herd Check IDEXX, Mastazyme MAST Diagnostics, P38-ELISA Animal Welfare and Food

Safety GmbH (AFOSA)) as well as in-house assays (five ELISAs and one IFAT). Most tests showed a high level of agreement in the interpretation of the test results (positive or negative). A further distinct increase in agreement between tests was obtained after the application of standardised cut-offs offered by a two-graph receiver operating characteristic analysis. This procedure allows a standardised interpretation of results obtained with different tests used in independent, parallel seroepidemiological studies.

10.13   Summary

1. Questions that determine the usefulness of a clinical test include:
   - What is the precision of the test?
   - How accurate is the test?
   - How often do the test results impact on clinical decisions?
   - What are the cost, risks and acceptability of the test?
   - Do the test results improve clinical outcomes?
   - What is the impact of the test result on the owner?
2. The clinical profiles of the study groups must be representative of the target testing population.
3. Blinding of the investigator to the disease status and the test results is important, particularly with subjective tests.
4. Measuring intra- and inter-observer precision is important if the test is subjective.
5. A gold standard is necessary to measure the accuracy of the test.
6. The performance of a diagnostic test can be quantified and illustrated by sensitivity, specificity, ROC curves and likelihood ratios.
7. The performance of prognostic studies can be summarized using risk/hazard ratios.

10.14   References

Fletcher RH, Fletcher SW, Wagner EH (1996) *Clinical Epidemiology (The Essentials)*, 3rd edn, Williams and Wilkins, Baltimore, p 269.

Gardner IA, Greiner M (2006) Receiver-operator characteristic curves and likelihood ratios: improvements over traditional methods for the evaluation and application of veterinary pathology tests. *Vet. Clin. Path.* **35**(1), 8–17.

Gerritzen-Bruning MJ, van den Ingh TS, Rothuizen J (2006) Diagnostic value of fasting plasma ammonia and bile acid concentrations in the identification of portosystemic shunting in dogs. *J. Vet. Intern. Med.* **20**(1): 13–19.

Page RB, Scrivani PV, Dykes NL, Erb HN, Hobbs JM (2006) Accuracy of increased thyroid activity during pertechnetate scintigraphy by subcutaneous injection for diagnosing hyperthyroidism in cats. *Vet. Radiol. Ultrasound* **47**(2): 206–11.

Peek SF, Semrad S, McGuirk SM, Riseberg A, Slack JA, Marques F, Coombs D, Lien L, Keuler N, Darien BJ (2006) Prognostic value of clinicopathologic variables obtained at admission and effect of antiendotoxin plasma on survival in septic and critically ill foals. *J. Vet. Intern. Med.* **20**(3): 569–74.

Stokel T, Erb H (1998) The apo-enzyme content of aminotranferases in healthy and diseased domestic animals. *Vet. Clin. Path.* **27:** 71–8.

Swets JA (1988) Measuring the accuracy of diagnostic systems. *Science* **240**: 1285–93.

Tepsumethanon V, Wilde H, Meslin FX (2005) Six criteria for rabies diagnosis in living dogs. *J. Med. Assoc. Thai.* **88**(3): 419–22.

Vercruysse J, Geurden T, Peelaers I (2006) Development and Bayesian evaluation of an ELISA to detect specific antibodies to *Sarcoptes scabiei* var suis in the meat juice of pigs. *Vet. Rec.* **158**(15): 506–8.

von Blumroder D, Schares G, Norton R, Williams DJ, Esteban-Redondo I, Wright S, Bjorkman C, Frossling J, Risco-Castillo V, Fernandez-Garcia A, Ortega-Mora LM, Sager H, Hemphill A, van Maanen C, Wouda W, Conraths FJ (2004) Comparison and standardisation of serological methods for the diagnosis of *Neospora caninum* infection in bovines. *Vet. Parasitol.* **120**(1–2): 11–22.

10.15   Further reading

Ajetunmobi O (2002) Critical appraisal of studies on diagnostic tests. In: *Making Sense of Critical Appraisal*, Arnold, London, pp 69–84.

Fletcher RH, Fletcher SW, Wagner EH (1996) Diagnosis. In: *Clinical Epidemiology (The Essentials)*, 3rd edn, Williams and Wilkins, Baltimore, pp 43–74.

Hulley SB, Cummings SR, Browner WS, Grady DG, Newman TB (2007) Designing studies of medical tests. In: *Designing Clinical Research*, 3rd edn, Lippincott Williams and Wilkins, Philadelphia, pp 188–206.

Smith RD (2006) Evaluation of diagnostic tests. In: *Veterinary Clinical Epidemiology*, 3rd edn, CRC Press, London, pp 33–52.

Thrusfield M (2005) Diagnostic trials. In: *Veterinary Epidemiology*, 3rd edn, Blackwell Publishing, Oxford, pp 305–30.

10.16   MCQs

1   *What is the odds equivalent to a 20% probability?*

(a)   0.2
(b)   1:5
(c)   0.25
(d)   1:4

2   *Which of the following best defines the terms 'sensitivity' and 'specificity'?*

(a)   Sensitivity is the proportion of diseased animals with a positive result.
Specificity is the proportion of animals without the disease with a negative result.
(b)   Sensitivity is the proportion of animals without the disease with a negative result.
Specificity is the proportion of diseased animals with a positive result.
(c)   Sensitivity is the proportion of true positives testing negative for the disease.
Specificity is the proportion of true negatives testing positive for the disease.
(d)   Sensitivity is the ratio of the true positives to the true negatives.
Specificity is the inverse of the sensitivity.

3   *What does the likelihood ratio for a negative test result tell us?*

(a)   The likelihood of the animal being disease free, given a negative test result.
(b)   The likelihood of the animal being disease free, given a positive test result.
(c)   The likelihood of the animal having a disease, given a negative test result.
(d)   The likelihood of the animal having a disease, given a positive test result.

4 *How would you best use a diagnostic test with a high specificity but a low sensitivity?*

(a) To rule a diagnosis out.
(b) To rule a diagnosis in.

5 *Receiver operator curves are useful because:*

(a) they indicate the cut-off point with the least diagnostic error
(b) they indicate which is the most accurate test
(c) they indicate the sensitivity and specificity at a given cut-off point
(d) all of the above.

6 *Given the sensitivity and specificity but not the prevalence it is possible to calculate:*

(a) the predictive value of a positive test result
(b) the predictive value of a negative result
(c) the likelihood ratio of a test result
(d) the accuracy
(e) the incidence.

7 *Prevalence can be determined using:*

(a) a case-control design
(b) a cross-sectional study
(c) a randomized controlled trial
(d) a retrospective prognosis study
(e) a prospective prognosis study.

8 *Subjective tests using observers should:*

(a) measure intra-observer agreement
(b) measure inter-observer agreement
(c) measure the kappa statistic
(d) ensure the observer is blinded to the status of the participant
(e) all of the above.

9 *Tandem testing can measure:*

(a) the sensitivity of a test
(b) the specificity of a test
(c) which of two tests is the most accurate
(d) the prevalence of disease
(e) the predictive values of the tests.

10 *Bias may be introduced by:*

(a) not blinding the observer
(b) using unrepresentative study groups
(c) using analyses that have not been calibrated
(d) not including all the results in the analysis
(e) all of the above.

10.17   MCQ answers

1. (c) 0.25, (d) 1:4; 2. (a); 3. (a); 4. (c); 5. (d); 6. (c), (e); 7. (b); 8. (e); 9. (c); 10. (e)

11

DESIGNING QUESTIONNAIRES

Objectives

After reading this chapter readers should:

- understand the principles of creating good questionnaires
- be able to design and use questionnaires and interviews.

Table 11.1   Stages in questionnaire design.

Define aims of survey
Formulate hypothesis
Define variables to be measured
Design and administer pilot study
Define and select sample population
Design a pilot survey
Update and administer finalized survey
Enter data
Analyse data
Report results

11.1   Introduction

There is often some confusion surrounding the terms 'questionnaire' and 'survey'. Clearly a questionnaire is a data collection tool that can be used in a variety of clinical and epidemiological research designs, but not all surveys require the use of a questionnaire.

Preparing a good questionnaire is a complex process requiring careful consideration. It is all too easy to lose sight of the primary research question, fail to consider the practicalities of processing the data and create problems for the person completing the form. The questionnaire provides the primary data for the study and while it does not require much effort to produce a poor questionnaire, it is well worth the effort required to produce a good design that does not disadvantage the study from the outset.

Generally the use of questionnaires in the majority of veterinary clinical research will be for quantitative, empirical research where the research question can be answered by counting or measuring the answers provided by the subject. There are occasions when we don't have a narrowly defined research question and require an explorative questionnaire consisting of open questions. This type of research falls under the umbrella of qualitative research and is beyond the scope of this textbook. Further reading on this subject is included in the further reading section at the end of this chapter. A summary of the stages in questionnaire design is shown in Table 11.1.

11.2   Designing a good questionnaire

Our objective in writing a good questionnaire is to create a tool that will provide the maximum amount of good quality (accurate) data that enables us answer the primary research question that the study is designed to answer. In practical terms this means that we want all the forms we issue to be filled out and returned to us with 100% accuracy. We can only achieve this if we ensure that the subjects are both willing to respond and have no difficulties filling in the form.

In order to be willing to spend time we need to 'sell' the advantages of participating in the research, which is covered later in this chapter. The questionnaire should contain no unnecessary questions because every additional question adds to the work required from the subjects. Each question should be as simple as possible and every effort should be taken to reduce the effort required from the subjects. The final principle in good questionnaire design is to reduce the scope for inaccuracy. This may be achieved by assisting recall with lists of possible responses or by providing opportunities for subjects to indicate where they are uncertain of the response.

11.3   Designing good questions

Good questionnaires require good questions. The first and most important aspect of each question is 'Why is the question being asked?'. There should always be a rationale that comes directly from the main research question. Avoid the temptation to collect additional information just because the opportunity arises; during the course of questionnaire design our creative juices may start flowing and additional research questions may arise that may enhance the study. However, it is important to think the whole process through. What research question are you adding to the study? Does it fit in with the overall aims and objectives? How will you process the data in order to answer your new research question? Is this questionnaire the best way to address this additional research aim?

As each question is written it is valuable to consider the following stages in the subject's response when filling out the questionnaire:

- Will the subject understand the question? While jargon is a useful technical shorthand it may be opaque to a layperson.
- Where is the subject going to obtain the information to answer this question? We may be relying on memory recall but if we expect a farmer to refer to their movement records we need to warn them of this fact before they start answering the questions.
- How objective or subjective is the response required? Do the response options reflect appropriately the likely answers that the subject may provide? Objective responses are easier to answer and interpret.
- Are the response options clear and unambiguous?

A good question is designed to maximize the chance of getting good quality data, i.e. an answer that is the true answer. In order to achieve this we need to consider bias, reliability and validity:

- bias: Could the wording of the question influence the respondents' answers?
- reliability: Would we get the same answer if the question were repeated?
- validity: Does the question actually measure the factor being investigated?

Questions are classed as 'open' when there are no restrictions on the type of response that can be given or 'closed' if the response has to be chosen from a pre-set list of answers.

11.3.1   Open questions

Open questions are generally more applicable to qualitative research. Free-text responses (e.g. What sort of exercise does your dog receive?) require specialized skills to analyse and interpret. Where it might be considered appropriate to use an open question to determine the weight of an animal from a respondent, it is nearly always better to provide a closed question asking for an approximate weight (e.g. 'Tick one of the following weight categories: < 5 kg, 5–10 kg, 10–15 kg, 15–20 kg, 20–25 kg, > 25 kg'). Many of us would not know the exact weight of a pet animal, and if we asked an open question we might well receive inconsistent results (e.g. different units, different precision, etc.) that complicate the analysis. Even something like a date is sometimes better requested in a closed format. If we are only going to use the year then there is no point in receiving the month or day parts of the date, particularly if asking for the date of birth of an animal, which may not be known by the owner with great precision. Indeed, if it is not clear to the respondent/subject that only the year is required they might just write 'not known', rather than rack their brains for the right answer.

One good use for an open question valuable for almost all surveys is to provide the respondent with an opportunity to comment on the questionnaire itself. It can be particularly frustrating not to be able to vent one's spleen about what one considers a design flaw in the questionnaire, and it provides some valuable feedback. Furthermore a respondent may, as a result, be more inclined to return the form rather than just discarding it.

11.3.2   Closed questions

There are a number of different formats that can be used to ask closed questions. These include:

- checklists (tick any of the following options that apply)
- multiple-choice questions (tick the one option that best applies)
- rating questions (indicate the response from the scale provided)
- ranking questions (indicate the importance/priority of the options provided)

The principal danger of the closed question is the omission of an appropriate response. While in human clinical research the gender options of male or female may be sufficient, in veterinary research we have to remember to include the neutered options (or ask for the neutered status in a separate question). While it is always possible to add a supplementary open option (typically 'Other' together with a box labelled 'Please specify'), when there are a large number of other possibilities it adds disproportionately to our work at the data entry, data handling and analysis stages of the research.

11.3.3   Checklists

Checklists provide a simple method of quickly asking (and answering) a number of non-mutually exclusive yes/no questions. They can be intimidating to fill in when they come in a large block and there is a danger that respondents start filling them in automatically or decide that it is easier to tick none of the options. If an option is omitted then it may not be possible for the respondent to provide an answer. Each option will require a separate variable/field in the questionnaire database (this will be a binary or logical field containing a yes/no value).

11.3.4   Multiple choice questions

In these questions we attempt to obtain a single response from the two or more options provided. Even a simple yes/no question might cause problems if the respondent doesn't remember or doesn't know. Questions must be mutually exclu-

sive (i.e. no overlap) and jointly exhaustive (i.e. cover all possible responses). A common error is illustrated below:

How many calves are housed in each pen?

(a)   < 5
(b)   5–10
(c)   10–15
(d)   15–20
(e)   > 20

The problem here is that if the calves are housed in pens of 10 or of 15 this could be entered as either one of two possible options.

When designing the layout of the options for objective responses, such as the number of calves in a pen, the use of the obvious numerical order of the options is clearly appropriate. For more subjective responses (e.g. 'How much does your dog scratch?') some care must be taken in the response options as, depending on the question, respondents will tend to favour items at the top or middle of the list. It is also important not to overburden the respondent with too many options. Received opinion is that a maximum of 10 options is appropriate for questionnaires filled in by the respondent, and five options for questionnaires filled in by an interviewer during face-to-face or telephone interviews.

The results from each question will be stored in a single field/variable in the study database as a numeric code representing the option chosen.

11.3.5   Rating questions

These questions are often used to attempt to obtain a quantitative value for something a respondent would normally think of in linguistic terms. A good example of this is the Likert scale, in which the respondent is asked to indicate their level of agreement with a statement (e.g. Statement: The cost of veterinary treatment represents good value for money. Responses: strongly agree, agree, neither agree or disagree, disagree, strongly disagree). Other approaches that can be used include asking for a numerical

If there was a likelihood of urinary incontinence following surgery, how would you feel about this?
Please indicate on the scale below your response between the extremes of acceptability.

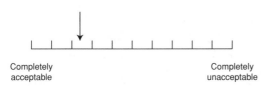

Completely acceptable   Completely unacceptable

Figure 11.1 An example of a visual analogue scale.

response (e.g. 'How satisfied are you with your veterinary treatment? Enter a number between 0 (dissatisfied) and 10 (satisfied)') or using a visual analogue scale (see Fig. 11.1). Many different variations have been used and compared in studies of questionnaire methodology and all of them have their faults. The biggest problem is the behavioural diversity of the people filling in the forms. Some personality types are reluctant to vary answers much from the neutral point while others veer between the extremes. There is also tremendous scope to bias the responses by sophisticated wording of the questions or statements, something that has long been exploited for political and marketing purposes. In designing a rating question consideration should be given to the number of options that are provided and whether or not there should be a neutral category. More than five to seven options is thought to help ensure the production of a continuous variable (as opposed to a series of categories). It may also be advisable to provide an option for respondents to indicate a failure to respond (don't know or don't have an opinion) that will distinguish these unanswered questions from other types of missing data.

Each answer will be stored as a single variable in the study database. If fewer than five options are provided these should be treated as ordinal data; if five or more options are provided then the answer can be treated as a continuous variable during analysis.

11.3.6 Ranking questions

These questions represent another attempt to obtain quantitative values about qualitative data. In a survey of client experience/satisfaction following cat neutering operations we might want to know how effectively we were communicating healthcare information. For example:

Please rank the following as sources of advice on the post-operative care and health information for your cat following its recent operation (1 = most useful or helpful information, 5 = least useful or helpful source).

Veterinarian
Veterinary nurse
Receptionist
Client advice leaflet
Practice website

It is quite important to avoid having too many options as it will then be difficult for the respondent to keep them in mind and simultaneously compare them. In face-to-face interviews the interviewer could hand the respondent a set of cards and ask for the cards back in order. The data handling and analysis of ranking questions can be problematic. Respondents may fail to rank items or duplicate ranks for two or more options (either deliberately or accidentally). The study design should include decisions about how to treat the data in these situations or to avoid the possibility through supervised questionnaire completion (e.g. in face-to-face or telephone interviews). Problems may also be avoided with careful programming of internet-based questionnaires.

Each option will be stored as a single ordinal variable in the study database. The ranks provided may not be equal (there is no option to indicate how much better or worse each option is) and it may be difficult to establish the most appropriate way to represent the cumulated results. An average rank (mean, median or mode) will be influenced by any missing data; it may be better to sum the number of respondents who ranked an option highly (e.g. 1 or 2) or higher than an option to which you want to compare it.

11.3.7 *Question wording*

As has already been suggested there is tremendous scope for introducing bias and reducing the quality of the responses through poorly worded questions.

One potential source of bias is to ask a leading question such as 'Should pain killers be used to reduce the suffering and discomfort of disbudding following the trauma of disbudding?'. A more neutral version of this question might be 'Should analgesics (non-steroidal drugs similar to aspirin and paracetamol/acetaminophen) be used following disbudding?'.

Avoid multiple questions leading to a single response. A question such as 'Is feline influenza a disease that you are concerned about that you believe should be vaccinated against?' addresses two issues at the same time. Respondents may have different views on the importance of the disease itself and the need for vaccination.

Lengthy questions or questions with an excessive preamble should be avoided. It has been suggested that questions should not be longer than 20 words. Lengthy questions will put off respondents and reduce compliance; furthermore there is a considerable risk that lengthy text will not be read or will be misread. Technical language, abbreviations and other jargon will also cause problems. A question such as 'Has your dog suffered from a GI problem in the last 12 months?' would be better worded as 'Has your dog suffered from an episode of diarrhoea or vomiting in the last 12 months?'.

11.4 Design and structure of the questionnaire forms

Where possible keep the design of the forms clear and simple. Avoid small type (less than 12pt) or excessive use of multiple typefaces (particularly ornamental typefaces). Careful use of highlighting such as italics, bold and increased point sizes may help, but avoid use of underlining and headings in capitals. Try to use white space (gaps between paragraphs and sections) to break up the text (white space around the margins is less important). Try to avoid multiple-page forms; an A3 sheet folded once to provide four pages of A4 won't intimidate most respondents whereas a block of 20 pages stapled together will seem overwhelming. Consider printing the form on coloured paper (preferably an inoffensive pastel shade); this will help respondents to locate the questionnaire if it ends up among a pile of other papers.

Although it is advisable to provide a covering letter explaining what the form is and why you would value a response, you should also provide some information on the form itself as the letter may well be discarded or become separated. There should also be clear instructions on how to complete the form. These instructions should contain an estimate of the length of time you think it will take to complete the questionnaire. Avoid separating instructions from the questions they apply to. For example, if one section of the form concerns the previous year and a following section the current year, this should be made clear on each of the two sections. People rarely read the instructions until they need help and it is preferable that they find this help on the same page that they encounter the problem. It may help to highlight the instructions by printing them in bold or italics.

It may be of benefit to provide instructions on how to return the completed questionnaire after the last question as a reminder that the questionnaire is of little value if it remains in the possession of the respondent. It is also worth thanking the respondent for their time.

Start off with simple straightforward questions. These help to build confidence and generate investment in the form (people are less likely to give up if they have already started).

Group the questions logically according to subject (e.g. breeding, housing, nutrition, etc.) or chronology (e.g. farrowing, weaning, fattening, finishing). If there are optional or conditional questions (i.e. answers that are only required if an animal has been neutered) then don't make respondents answer 'not applicable' to numerous irrelevant questions; make it clear that they can proceed to the next relevant question. Some caution is required when considering a branching structure to the questions as extra care will be required to avoid confusing the respondent. Simple linear structures may be preferable if the questionnaire is relatively short. Providing structure within a section, for example moving from easily answered questions to more detailed questions on the same subject, helps to prompt the respondent's memory. Consider carefully how a respondent may be able to answer questions; if appropriate ask them to refer to records (but remember to warn them in the preamble). Some care may be required to avoid prior questions influencing subsequent questions. If an unbiased response to the question 'Would you vaccinate your animal?' is required it would be foolish to precede it with a section which either explicitly or implicitly focused the respondent's mind on the consequences of the disease in question.

11.5 Reply-paid envelope

The provision of a correctly addressed reply-paid envelope is both a courtesy and tool that may help to increase response rates. The use of a reply-paid service will ensure that only those envelopes that are used are paid for.

11.6 The covering letter

However the questionnaire is delivered, some sort of explanation should be provided to the respondent to justify the investment in their time and effort. The information given here on the covering letter applies equally to the preamble required for direct interviews, telephone interviews and internet-based surveys.

The covering letter should provide the following information:

- Who you are
- The purpose of the survey
- The main areas covered in the survey
- How long the survey will take to fill in
- Why you have selected the addressee/respondent
- Assurance of data confidentiality
- Instructions on how to return the questionnaire
- A thank you

Generally compliance is greater when responses are elicited from recognized educational or scientific institutions such as a university department or university veterinary hospital; if one of the research team has a legitimate association with such an institution it may well be possible to use an official letterhead and their postal address.

Explaining why and how you obtained the respondent's personal details is not only a basic courtesy, it may also help to legitimize the survey if it indicates concrete support from a breed society or a trade association.

In assuring data confidentiality some consideration should be given to how much sensitive information is required and the practicality of upholding those assurances. If the questionnaire hopes to obtain sensitive personal information (e.g. financial data) then a completely anonymous questionnaire is much more likely to be returned and there will be a bias in the personality type who respond. This also has the disadvantage that it is then not possible to chase up non-responders or to follow up groups of responders for follow-up surveys. It this is a major issue it may be worth using an intermediate organization (such as the Electoral Reform Society in the UK) who may be prepared to administer the personalized information and pass on individualized data (e.g. replacing names with identification numbers) and thus assure anonymity to the respondents. In any event the response rates will be improved by the assurance that the data will only be used for the purposes laid out in the letter.

Clearly a postal address for the return of the completed questionnaire should be provided both in the letter and on the form. Ideally a reply-paid envelope should be provided, as mentioned above, which can be arranged with a variety of postal services in most countries.

Every attempt should be made to keep the covering letter short and clear; ideally it should be kept to a single page. Using the mail-merge facilities available with most word processors and databases it is relatively simple to personalize covering letters. This helps to reinforce the belief in the respondent that the research is directed specifically to the respondent and that they are not just receiving a broadly directed mailing.

11.7   Pilot testing

The more people who get a chance to comment on the questionnaire design before it is sent out to real respondents the better. Start with members of the research team but also include a wide variety of non-veterinarians, non-researchers and lay people; they may produce some irrelevant comments but are often able to spot hidden pitfalls that would otherwise be missed.

A formal pilot testing stage is highly desirable. This provides an opportunity to test the questionnaire on a sample of the actual population of respondents. It may be worth adding some specific questions on the questionnaire design itself at this stage. The pilot study will provide an early indication of response rates and this, together with any power calculations that have been performed, will indicate how many questionnaires will need to be sent out. It will also provide some test data to test the data handling and analysis procedures to be used in the study.

The responses to each question should be examined. Does the variety in responses correspond to what might reasonably be expected? Is the distribution of values appropriate? Are any of the questions being asked producing an excessive number of null responses or consistently producing an identical response (where a variety of responses might be expected)? This information will help to identify problematic questions and provide an opportunity to improve their wording or format.

11.8   Maximizing response

Studies affected by low response rates will be underpowered. This means that the statistical confidence in any results obtained will be reduced and any biasing factors are likely to influence these results. A study by Edwards et al. (2002) looked at a large number of surveys performed in medical research to identify any factors that may affect the response rates to questionnaires. Some of their findings are listed below; the figures in brackets are the confidence intervals of the odds ratios.

11.8.1   *Positive factors*

- Relevance of questionnaire to participant (1.99–3.01)
- Questionnaire design:
  - short questionnaire (1.55–2.24)
  - personalized (1.06–1.28)
  - coloured ink (1.16–1.67)
- Advance warning of survey (1.34–1.92)
- Reminders (1.22–1.70)
- Monetary incentive (1.79–2.27)
- Origin: university vs other organization (1.11–1.54)

11.8.2   *Negative factors*

- Sensitive question included (0.87–0.98)
- Choice to opt out (0.65–0.89)

If low response rates are identified as a problem these factors may be considered. If the sensitivity of the data is likely to be a problem then anonymous responses might be considered. The method of administration of the questionnaire

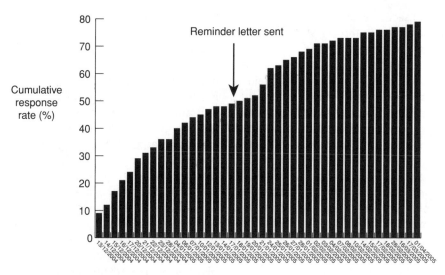

Figure 11.2 A graph showing the effect of a follow-up letter during a survey sent to organizers of agricultural shows in the UK.

may also help to reduce or address low response rates (see below).

11.9 Follow-up letters

As part of the initial study design of a postal questionnaire the value of a reminder letter should be considered. This may be directed at identified non-responders or the full mailing list in the case of an anonymous response survey.

The reminder letter should re-emphasize the purpose of the survey, the importance of their response in reducing bias and any promise of confidentiality of the information provided. It may be desirable to identify responses resulting from the follow-up. This can be achieved by adding a new question to the re-sent questionnaire or a subtle formatting change. This won't be an absolute measure of the response to the follow-up letter as the reminder will often lead to the respondent retrieving the original form and returning that one. The effect of a follow-up letter during a survey sent to organizers of agricultural shows is shown in Fig. 11.2.

11.10 Administration of the questionnaire

Questionnaires can be administered in a number of ways. This chapter has focused primarily on the use of questionnaires in a postal survey but they may also be administered by direct face-to-face interviews, telephone interviews and internet-based forms on websites.

Postal questionnaires are relatively cheap to distribute to respondents over a wide geographical area. They can be filled out at a time convenient to the respondent and respondents can be relatively confident of their anonymity. However, the response rates are typically quite low on postal surveys and the speed of return is highly variable. Illegible handwriting may have an impact on the ease of data entry and the quality of the data.

Face-to-face interviews are affected by the additional factor of the interviewer themselves. Respondents will be less inclined to answer personal questions and may be inclined to give what they consider to be more socially acceptable responses. When there are lots of conditional questions (e.g. subsidiary questions based on the response to earlier questions giving a branching structure to the questionnaire) this is handled by the interviewer and avoids challenging the respondent with a highly complex paper form. The quality of the data obtained from an interview are dependent on the training and diligence of the interviewer, and variation of interviewer quality may affect the quality of the study data. Face-to-face interviews are expensive to perform but give the researcher more control over the completion of the questionnaire. They are particularly useful in situations where there are relatively few potential respondents and therefore high response rates are essential (e.g. a follow-up survey for an uncommon veterinary procedure carried out at a referral centre).

Telephone interviews have similar advantages and disadvantages to face-to-face interviews. There is an increasing resistance to responding to unsolicited telephone calls as a result of their misuse by commercial organizations. It may be worth paving the way with an introductory letter and giving respondents the opportunity to specify when they would be prepared to provide time for the interview. This enables a more efficient use of the interviewer's time and avoids the problem of travel if the respondents are distributed over a wide geographical area.

The main advantage of the internet-based questionnaire is the saving in data-handling costs. Website forms can be constructed so that the information is directly entered into the study database. Computerized forms also have the advantage that basic data errors can be caught as the information is entered (e.g. an invalid date, text in a response where a number is required, etc.); they can also automatically handle branching forms with subsidiary questions. There is major potential for bias in that both access to, and a willingness to use, a computer is not evenly distributed among the population. It may be worth considering providing a website address as an alternative to a paper-based questionnaire but allowing either to be used. Internet-based questionnaires are particularly valuable when a large number of respondents are being approached. There may be a tendency for more casual or careless data entry by some respondents when faced with long forms. It is very important that the respondent is given a clear indication of how much work is required and that feedback is provided on progress through the form (respondents may give up if they get bored and don't realize that there are only a couple of questions to go before they would have finished). The quality of the design and programming is vital, which makes these questionnaires expensive and difficult to set up. They need to be tested exhaustively using every permutation that the most deranged individual might possibly attempt. Some of the best testers are students given the challenge of 'breaking' the questionnaire system.

11.11 Validation

Questionnaires and their questions should be assessed for validity (roughly equivalent to accuracy) and for reproducibility (precision) in the same way that any diagnostic test might be examined (see Chapter 10).

The first step is to consider the face validity of each question. This is a subjective judgement on whether the question asks what you think it is asking. This judgement should be repeated by as many external, impartial observers as can be coerced into providing help.

Is there a gold standard to which the results from pilot testing can be compared? This may be obtained from other relevant sets of data or through the simultaneous collection of the same data through other instruments (e.g. are the distributions of age, sex and breed of animals similar to those found in comparable populations?). There are clearly practical limitations on ensuring the accuracy of responses. As with any clinical research study, thought should be given to the ultimate value in being able to assess the absolute accuracy and the potential legitimate criticism of any interpretation of the results that may arise from lack of confidence in the accuracy of the primary data. Ultimately the predictive validity of the data obtained can be assessed by its ability to correlate future outcomes from any associations revealed by the original questionnaire.

Within the survey population it may be deemed necessary to re-test a subsample with a different instrument to look at the repeatability of the responses. The use of more than one question to obtain the same information is one way of doing this. However, before such steps are taken the researcher should consider what they would do with the information obtained. It is clearly valuable to quantify the repeatability of responses giving a lameness score when veterinarians are shown videos of lame animals. On the other hand, asking owners for both the date of birth and the age of their pets may serve to annoy the more numerate respondents, and what value is it to the researcher to quantify the difference in ages derived from different questions in the absence of a gold standard?

11.12　How things can go wrong

Most of the potential disasters have already been alluded to in the sections above. Errors will always occur due to the intrinsic variability in the natural world. We ameliorate or minimize the potential of these errors to invalidate our research through careful design and exhaustive testing of the questionnaires. Expect there to be problems, anticipate what they might be and plan for them.

Common sources of problems are respondent errors due to misinterpretation of questions, a lack of interest in the survey, unwillingness to admit to certain behaviour and poor memory recall. Interview-administered questionnaires may be impaired as a result of interview stress, pressure on time and interviewer error. Respondents may consistently fail to respond to certain questions for a variety of rea-

sons and it may be difficult for the researcher to work out why this occurs; sometimes a simple re-wording of the question can be of help.

At the study design level a low response rate can severely damage the power of the study and introduce significant bias. A failure to anticipate sources of bias or confounding factors can be a major problem when attempting to interpret the results. It can be extremely frustrating to realize after the questionnaire results have been collated that it is not possible to test for a potential confounder when the information could have been easily collected by a simple additional question. One further pitfall that should be addressed at the design stage and tested in a pilot phase is data processing. Failure to anticipate data entry, handling and analysis requirements can prevent a promising study from progressing beyond the administration of the questionnaire. An additional aspect of the questionnaire design is the inclusion and formatting of the form to optimize data entry. Prior to data entry there should also be procedures in place to deal with ambiguous or illegible responses.

11.13　Reference

Edwards P, Roberts I, Clarke M, DiGuiseppi C, Pratap S, Wentz R, Kwan I (2002) Increasing response rates to postal questionnaires: systematic review. *BMJ* **324**: 1183.

11.14　Further reading

Dohoo I, Martin W, Stryhn H (2003) Questionnaire design. In: *Veterinary Epidemiologic Research*, AVC Inc., Charlottestown, Prince Edward Island, pp 53–64.
Hulley SB, Cummings SR, Browner WS, Grady DG, Newman TB (2007) Designing questionnaires and data collection instruments. In: *Designing Clinical Research*, 3rd edn, Lippincott Williams and Wilkins, Philadelphia, pp 241–255.
Kumar R (2005) Selecting a method of data collection. In: *Research Methodology*, 2nd edn, Sage Publications, London, pp 126–42.

Labaw PJ (1980) *Advanced Questionnaire Design*, Abt Books, Cambridge, Massachusetts.

Oppenheim AN (1992) *Questionnaire Design, Interviewing and Attitude*, Continuum, New York.

Thrusfield M (2005) Data collection and management. In: *Veterinary Epidemiology*, 3rd edn, Blackwell Publishing, Oxford, pp 188–95.

11.15   MCQs

1   **Which of the following type of question is an open question?**

(a)   Checklists.
(b)   Multiple-choice.
(c)   Rating questions.
(d)   Ranking questions.
(e)   Numerical entry.

2   **What is a Likert scale?**

(a)   A measure of how good a question is.
(b)   A type of question asking how strongly a respondent agrees or disagrees with a statement.
(c)   A question where the respondent is asked how strongly they agree with a statement on a scale of 1 to 10.
(d)   A type of open question.
(e)   A question to which the respondent answers 'Yes' or 'No'.

3   **Which of the following should not be included in a covering letter?**

(a)   The purpose of the survey.
(b)   Personal details of other people being surveyed.
(c)   How long the survey will take to fill in.
(d)   Why you have selected the addressee/ respondent.
(e)   Instructions on how to return the questionnaire.

4   **Which of the following are useful in arriving at a final design for a questionnaire?**

(a)   Fixing clear survey objectives.
(b)   Showing the draft design to colleagues.
(c)   Repeating questions with different wordings.
(d)   Pilot testing the questionnaire.
(e)   Using ornamental fonts.

5   **Which of the following are positive factors in maximizing the response to a questionnaire?**

(a)   Short questionnaire.
(b)   Personalized form.
(c)   Coloured ink.
(d)   Choice to opt out.
(e)   Advance warning of survey.

6   **Which of the following are negative factors in maximizing the response to a questionnaire?**

(a)   Relevance of questionnaire to participant.
(b)   Sensitive question included.
(c)   Monetary incentive.
(d)   Choice to opt out.
(e)   Reminders.

7   **Which of the following is not a technique that can be used to help validate the data from a questionnaire?**

(a)   Simultaneous collection of data through another instrument.
(b)   Comparing data from that collected in other studies or populations.
(c)   Re-testing a subsample.
(d)   Asking respondents to sign the questionnaire.
(e)   Checking that the result is the one expected.

11.16   MCQ answers

1. (e); 2. (b); 3. (b); 4. (a), (b) and (d); 5. (a), (b), (c) and (e); 6. (b) and (d); 7. (d)

12

STUDY
IMPLEMENTATION

Objectives

After reading this chapter readers should:

- appreciate the need to consider quality control
- be able to implement appropriate quality control strategies
- understand pilot studies and pre-testing.

12.1   Pilot studies and pre-testing

There are two obvious situations when pilot studies are clearly indicated. Firstly, when the study is working in an area where there is no previously published data. In this case the pilot study will provide essential information for sample size calculations and may be required to provide information on the basic feasibility of the project. The second clear indication for a pilot study is when the size or scale of the project involves a large number of subjects or an effort from a large number of people. In this case even a minor problem may lead to a lot of wasted effort or a considerable financial expense and a pilot study is readily justified by the potential cost saving.

Short of a full pilot study some form of pre-testing is always advisable. The value of pre-testing in studies using questionnaires has been described in Chapter 11 but all studies will benefit from some degree of pre-testing. Appropriate members of the team (i.e. some of the staff who will need to use them) should check the documentation. Sampling techniques, labels, data entry forms and analysis procedures are all worth trying out before the study begins. While there is considerable intellectual satisfaction in the design and initial planning of a research project, it is the attention to the practical details that makes the biggest contribution to success or failure, even if this is the boring bit.

A pre-testing phase provides an opportunity to rehearse the research team. There is a need for clearly written documentation containing instructions for all members of the team, and for the information and education of all participants, but these documents don't provide the opportunity for questions. Running a dress rehearsal as a training exercise will provide an opportunity for those involved to raise any problems and possibly suggest minor modifications. It should also help to provide some consistency in the application of techniques, particularly if there are varying levels of experience among the clinicians or technical staff involved.

At the very least it is worth reviewing progress after data from the first few subjects have been collected. Ideally the research team should meet and review the procedures that have been used and receive confirmation that the data collected are in the format that was expected. This will also provide some feedback on any problems encountered.

12.2   Quality control

A further unheralded but nonetheless important area for consideration before the main study starts is quality control. There is a feeling that once data collection has commenced the project is on course and little further work needs to be done until all the data have arrived for processing.

12.2.1   Missing data

If there are missing data from a large proportion of subjects the whole study can be wrecked, and even a relatively few missing values can lead to exclusions that introduce significant bias. Some missing data should be anticipated at the design phase and decisions made on how these subjects will be treated during analysis.

The first approach should be to monitor the data as they are collected. Sometimes the missing value can be readily retrieved if its absence is detected early enough and often the animal or client can be recalled (with apologies) to enable a sample to be re-taken.

Extended follow-up periods present particular problems because dropouts may be biased as a result of loss of communication with clients. While the client may be particularly happy with the outcome of treatment and sees no particular need to return for yet another re-evaluation, they may have forgotten or may not realize the importance of this fact being recorded. This may lead to significant bias when less successful outcomes are over-represented.

There are some statistical techniques that may be used to provide missing values (under the guidance of a statistician) but, as ever, prevention is better than cure. These techniques are particularly useful in the case of multivariate analysis to avoid the exclusion of too many subjects due to the accumulation of missing data across a number of predictor variables.

12.2.2   *Inaccurate and imprecise data*

Variations in the precision and accuracy of data constitute an insidious problem that may remain a hidden cause of the poor performance of a study (see Chapter 4). Inevitably there are differences between veterinary clinicians, laboratories, machines, etc. Potential problems should be anticipated at the design phase, particularly where relatively subjective clinical assessments are being made (e.g. lameness). Consistency in laboratory results or where machinery is used can be checked during the study using standard samples or repeated samples.

The problem is all the worse when it is not detectable. While the placebo effect is less of a significant factor in veterinary research it is still evident in studies that use clients/owners to assess their animals' health. If the trial is inadvertently unblinded unbeknownst to the investigator, this may lead to the drawing of incorrect conclusions from the trial results.

12.2.3   *Fraudulent data*

Quite apart from outright intentional deception we have to face the reality of laziness, carelessness and simple human error. Our first approach

should be to emphasize the need for integrity and the second approach is to make all tasks as easy as possible to perform correctly. A good working relationship with motivated staff who have some 'ownership' of the project helps to establish a code of ethical behaviour which is reinforced by their involvement at the planning stage rather than just using them as labour. Pre-printed labels and well-designed forms all help with the ergonomics of boring and repetitive tasks.

Establish a culture of responsibility rather than blame. Staff can often help to establish good cross-checking procedures for avoiding mix-ups during sample or data collection. Errors are less likely to occur when working as a pair or in a team. Establishing a protocol that reconfirms important identification data before an animal is returned to its owner or back to a pen will help to reduce problems. The use of automated identification systems such as transponders or microchips can be useful when ear-tag numbers or freeze brands are difficult to read. All of these approaches will help to avoid the temptation to provide 'guessed at' data to cover up a mistake.

A further check on fraudulent data entry is to require members of the research team to maintain all hand-written records in a hard-bound notebook or ring binder rather than asking them to fill in the results in a computerized record such as a spreadsheet or database. Although the computerized record will be required for analysis, it is relatively easy to edit while the paper record will provide less disputable evidence.

12.2.4   *Randomization*

Using inappropriate randomization methods that are arbitrary in nature, rather than truly random, may introduce bias inadvertently. Consider the sampling of dairy cows as they pass through the milking parlour. The more dominant or confident cows tend to push to the front of queue and the in-parlour feeding system may be more generous on one side of the parlour when compared to the other. If the herd is divided into two by the order they come through to be milked, or on the basis of which side of the parlour they are milked on, the sampling will be biased. The only truly random method of sampling is to use an independent selection on the basis of chance. This can involve a random number sequence generated by a computer (this is easily done using a spreadsheet program), selecting numbers/names from a hat or even throwing dice. Proper randomization takes very little effort to perform properly; it eliminates sampling bias and inspires confidence in the reader (or reviewer) that the research has been performed properly.

12.2.5   Quality control of clinical and laboratory procedures

These quality control tools will be prepared during the planning phase of the study and should be reviewed throughout the data collection phase.

The operations manual

For each clinical or laboratory procedure a clear set of instructions will be required. This will be an expanded practical version of the methods section of the protocol. It should be written in language that is suitable for a wide background of educational levels as appropriate for the readership. The operations manual is of particular importance when the procedure is to be carried out at different clinics with different staff to ensure consistency. It should not assume any prior knowledge about the trial but should be clearly structured to ensure that any information can be quickly found and assimilated by the reader.

Training

Staff participating in the trial should be adequately qualified for the procedures that they are expected to perform. It is also important that they have relevant experience that ensures they are capable of performing the tasks involved competently and consistently. It may be necessary to provide training for new machinery or techniques and for newly acquired skills to be tested or assessed.

Some training is essential where staff are to be involved in helping owners, clients or animal carers to fill out questionnaires. While the collection of small amounts of objective information may not be influenced by the attitude or personal skills of the interviewer, the completion of more extensive questionnaires can be seriously affected by untrained or poorly trained staff (see Chapter 11).

Leadership and supervision

Veterinary clinical research is almost inevitably a team exercise and leadership skills will contribute to the overall performance of the team. Over-solicitous supervision may generate resentment, while appropriate delegation will provide responsibility and independence, resulting in a feeling of ownership. Effective and regular communication and the acknowledgement of the contribution of all the team members will help maintain motivation.

Research staff meetings

Appropriate meetings in person, by telephone or using the internet should be included in the study design. As with the pre-testing phase they provide an opportunity to identify and solve problems. They are potentially a good source of boosting morale and generating interest in the goals of the study when staff can see progress being made and their contribution to it.

Periodic reviews

Communication of intermediate results both internally and externally is a valuable tool to encourage compliance and assist with recruitment. It may not be possible to provide interim results but a progress report and a restatement of the value of the study may prompt a more timely or considered completion of a questionnaire. For participating colleagues, updates on the quality of information or minor problems others have had can focus their attention on the continued need for careful compliance. At the very least it lets everyone know that the study has not died.

A formal review may be included in a large project as part of a formal quality control process. The review may be performed by independent experts who have access to unblinded data to provide an opportunity to examine interim results. Building this level of scrutiny into the study design may help to reassure funding bodies who are being asked to provide substantial financial support.

Quality control coordinator

In a large study it may be advisable to assign the responsibility for quality control to a single individual. This individual can be allowed a degree of autonomy and independence in the examination of records and study results. While a spot check from the quality control coordinator will not be a welcome event, the knowledge that it might happen can be a strong motivator.

Blinding

The value of blinding has already been described in the chapters on study design. While the rationale for blinding clinicians and owners is relatively obvious, the rationale for the blinding of objective measurements carried out in external laboratories may be less clear. Firstly, if every aspect is kept blind at all possible stages then there is less chance of the blinding being accidentally revealed. Secondly, the blinding process makes it easier to include additional samples such as duplicates and standard samples. On a practical level it helps to allocate this job to a member of the team, such as the quality control supervisor, who has no responsibilities for collecting, recording, interpreting or analysing

data. This person is then responsible for holding the keys or codes that 'unblind' the trial at the end of the analysis phase. There should also be a contingency plan, for example lodging the blinding information in a sealed envelope with a third party, in case the chosen person should be unavailable when the information is required.

Sample labelling, storage and handling

Nothing is more depressing than discovering that samples have been lost due to coagulation, contamination, leakage, damage to containers or loss of labelling. The clinical samples are often the most essential component of a study. Do not economize on expenditure in this area. Compared to the cost of the human effort involved, the cost of storage is minimal. Purchase the highest quality containers and labels that are guaranteed not to come unstuck when wet or frozen. Generally pre-printed labels are preferable; they save time and are almost certainly more legible than most clinicians' handwriting. Storing duplicate or multiple sets of aliquotted samples in different locations in case samples are lost or contaminated is a backup procedure akin to backing up data on a computer. Freezers may break down, samples can be accidentally discarded and problems may occur in external laboratories. Having an extra set of samples is an excellent form of insurance.

12.2.6 Quality control of data

Consideration of the data management of results is described in Chapter 13 and should form part of the study design phase. All aspects should be implemented and tested before any data are collected, including any paper forms, electronic forms and databases.

Form designs

As has been described above, good ergonomic design and ensuring that questionnaires are not excessively long are great aids to quality assurance. Forms should be designed in conjunction with the database to force the investigator to provide accurate standardized responses. The majority of form design issues are covered in Chapter 11.

Data that involve judgement will need explicit operational definitions that are summarized on the form itself and explained in more detail in the operations manual. The sections should be laid out in a logical fashion consistent with the likely sequence in which the data will be collected. Avoid asking for any data that have already been collected. If the subject has already been assigned a number it may be useful to ask for confirmation of name and postcode as a quality control measure but the re-entry of a complete address is redundant if that information has already been collected.

Data checking and entry

If the data collected can be manually checked before the animal and the client leave the building this allows for correction of errors or collection of missing data with a minimum of fuss. Ideally this should be performed by another team member and might be achieved by including a final check as part of the discharge procedure performed by lay staff.

An important data-checking opportunity comes when the information is entered in the computer records. All databases allow for some level of error detection when data are input. The data entry screen can be programmed to flag up inconsistent entries, missing values and parameters that are out of the expected range. The sophistication of this error checking will depend on the size of the study and effort the investigators feel it is worth making. Further guidance on data handling is covered in Chapter 13.

Reviewing the data

An examination of the values of important parameters may be carried out periodically to give an indication of the frequency distribution and identify any outliers (very high or very low values). This may help to identify obvious problems with individual data sets or more systematic problems (e.g. an absence of any subjects in an important category). These reviews should be performed as early as possible to ensure that there is still time to address any problems revealed (e.g. when it is still possible to recall an animal for resampling or re-examination).

12.2.7   Multi-site studies

All of the potential problems with quality control are exacerbated when more than one veterinary clinic or hospital is involved in the study. Problems can only be avoided through meticulous planning, thorough organization and good communication. The need and value of research team meetings is increased and it may be worth considering an overall governance panel with some external or independent members to assist in resolving any conflicts. In veterinary clinical research studies are rarely so large that this is required. The vast majority of problems arise from misunderstandings and miscommunication.

12.3   Revising the protocol once the study has begun

It is inevitable that there will be some alterations in the precise protocol that is actually implemented. It would obviously be foolish to adhere to a flawed protocol, but as a rule changes to the protocol should be kept to a minimum.

12.3.1   Minor revisions to the protocol

The majority of minor protocol changes involve modifications to the operations manual. A change in the gauge of needle used to take a sample to speed up the time taken or clarification of an exclusion criterion due to circumstances that hadn't been anticipated are typical examples of such modifications. These changes are unlikely to affect the data collected. Once a decision has been made the important thing is firstly to amend the protocol, including the reasons for the change. Secondly, any documents affected, such as the operations manual, should be amended. Lastly, and most importantly, the decision should be communicated to the entire research team.

Changes that are likely to influence the quality or nature of the data are more problematic. If a questionnaire is altered to include a response that was not previously present on the form, the data collected using the original questionnaire will be materially different from the new questionnaire. A decision to make the change may clearly be needed but there are then problems associated with the analysis of that data. If relatively little data has been collected the change may have no effect on the result. It may be that the change was triggered by a significant number of respondents providing the information as an 'other' response and the change is purely to improve the ergonomics of the form. Each case must be treated on its own merits and good statistical advice can often help to minimize any detrimental effect on the overall study results.

12.3.2   Substantial revisions to the protocol

More substantive changes to the protocol, such as changing the intervention, an outcome measure used or the population from which the animals are taken, are likely to present a more serious problem. The recruitment of cases may have been much lower than was originally anticipated and so either a less proscriptive case definition is employed or animals from more than one location are included. Clearly there is no point in continuing with a trial that has proved not to be feasible using the existing protocol. A subjective judgement will be made as to the likelihood that this will have a major effect on the results. In these cases the uniformity of the study population will be reduced, leading to the possibility of a greater number of potential confounding factors and also an increase in the variance of

the output measure that will reduce the power of the study.

If a substantial body of data has been collected then it may be possible to deal with this at the analysis stage by considering the pre- and post-protocol change subjects as two separate groups. A statistical examination of the two sets of data will provide some indication of the best analysis strategy to use. It should be possible to recalculate the sample size and include this in the protocol revision to ensure that data are collected from sufficient animals to produce a meaningful result.

In the worst case scenario, and particularly if data have been collected from relatively few animals, the best option is to treat the work completed as a pilot study and to start the main study again.

12.4   Further reading

Dohoo I, Martin W, Stryhn H (2003) A structured approach to data analysis. In: *Veterinary Epidemiologic Research*, AVC Inc., Charlottestown, Prince Edward Island, pp 581–90.

Hulley SB, Cummings SR, Browner WS, Grady DG, Newman TB (2007) Implementing the study: pretesting, quality control and protocol revisions. In: *Designing Clinical Research*, 3rd edn, Lippincott Williams and Wilkins, Philadelphia, pp 271–89.

Pocock SJ (1983) Protocol deviations. In: *Clinical Trials: A Practical Approach*, John Wiley and Sons, Chichester, pp 176–86.

12.5   MCQs

1 *Pilot studies offer which of the following advantages?*

(a) They enable pilot data to be collected for sample size estimation.

(b) They enable data collection and entry systems to be rehearsed.

(c) They identify potential practical problems with data collection.

(d) They can provide estimates of likely client compliance.

(e) They help to indicate the likely duration of the trial.

2 *Which of the following may not have an adverse effect on the quality of the data collected in a study?*

(a) Poor training of staff.
(b) Missing data.
(c) Fraudulent data.
(d) Good study documentation and operations manuals.
(e) Relying on hand-written notes.

3 *Which of the following can be used to protect against fraud?*

(a) Periodic monitoring of staff and data.
(b) The maintenance of hand-written notebooks or journals.
(c) Working in pairs or teams.
(d) Appointing a quality control supervisor.
(e) Requiring staff to sign a non-disclosure agreement.

4 *Which of the following strategies helps to improve the quality of the data?*

(a) Well-designed forms.
(b) Appointing a quality control supervisor.
(c) Periodically reviewing the data.
(d) Implementing a data-checking protocol.
(e) Getting a second member of staff to check data immediately after they have been entered.

5 *How should minor changes to the study protocols be handled?*

(a) Give staff discretion to makes changes they feel are necessary.
(b) Only allow supervisors to make changes when necessary.
(c) Allow changes to be made but make sure operations manuals are updated.
(d) When changes are made, make a careful record of why the change was made and what changes were made.
(e) No changes to the protocol should ever be allowed.

6 *How should major changes to the protocol not be handled?*

(a) No substantial changes to the protocol should ever be allowed.
(b) Restart the study using the revised protocol.
(c) Analyse the data using the different protocols separately.
(d) Treat the data collected before the protocol change as a pilot study .
(e) Continue the study but increase the sample size.

7 *Which of the following is the best method of blinding the laboratory analysis of samples?*

(a) Leave all data labelled but use an independent laboratory.
(b) Ask the laboratory to blind the samples.
(c) Send the samples from different groups to different laboratories.
(d) Pre-label sample pots using a numeric code giving no indication of the animal's identity or group.
(e) Send a duplicate set of samples to a second laboratory.

8 *Which of the following methods is most suitable for randomizing animals to intervention groups?*

(a) Putting alternate animals in the two different groups.
(b) Taking the animal's name and allocating them to groups on the basis of the first letter of their name.
(c) Using the day of the week that the animal was sampled to determine their group.
(d) Throwing a dice to determine group allocation.
(e) Asking the owner which group they would like their animal to be in.

12.6 MCQ answers

1. All the options describe the potential advantages of a pilot study; 2. (d); 3. (e); 4. All the options describe strategies to improve the quality of data; 5. (d) It is also important to revise all operational documents; 6. (e); 7. (d); 8. (d)

13

DATA MANAGEMENT

Objectives

After reading this chapter readers should:

• understand the basic requirements for the effective storage and use of data.

13.1   General considerations

The need to be well organized and disciplined has already been conveyed in previous chapters. Smaller veterinary studies are generally the work of a single individual, albeit with the help of other essential team members. Some of us are naturally well organized, but others of us (and particularly this author) require considerable self-discipline to maintain our records in good order. During the training research students receive the need to maintain a laboratory notebook is emphasized. This takes the form of a log or diary in which every detail of the planning and execution of experiments is meticulously recorded. This enables us to return to what was done and decided on after the event to help with the eventual writing up of the work and in the resolution of problems that subsequently come to light. It is strongly recommended that this approach is also adhered to for clinical research projects. If, like the author, you are not well organized, the use of a hardback notebook is preferred to a loose-leaf binder. Loose documents may be pasted into a notebook or included in sections of a binder. In any event notes should be kept of meetings, copies of the relevant literature (or lists of references), pilot data, contact details, etc. In this way, different versions of operational documents and revision lists can be referred to when necessary. It is also worth remembering that the paper copies of documents that are held on computers represent the ultimate technology-free backup solution.

13.2   Computing requirements

While it is perfectly feasible for a veterinary clinical research project to be completed without the use of a computer, the acquisition of basic computer literacy will make a massive difference to the amount of work involved. While some of our greatest creative writers may eschew the use of a word processor, many of the rest of us cannot imagine attempting to write more than a few lines without the editing facilities provided by our computers.

When it comes to managing the data generated by a study the spreadsheet (e.g. Microsoft Excel) provides an indispensable tool that is the equivalent of using a word processor to manage text. Even if the manipulation and analysis are subsequently going to be performed by a third party using a different computer package the spreadsheet is an excellent tool to use and almost all other computer programs can read information that is stored in a spreadsheet format, providing some care has been taken with the layout and entry of the data.

If the investigator is prepared to develop their spreadsheet skills to a basic level it will be possible for them to perform all basic statistical analyses using a spreadsheet. These skills are often best learnt from performing real tasks rather than attempting to plough through the instruction manual. However, do not wait until the data collection phase is completed before first attempting to process the data and using a spreadsheet for the first time. Using a spreadsheet to manage your personal finances or budgeting for a holiday are good exercises to learn how the spreadsheet program works. Calculating means and standard variations of small sets of pilot data will provide a good introduction to the basic statistical functions and subsequently pave the way for performing power calculations to estimate sample size. When some basic data-handling tasks have been performed some of the common problems, errors and limitations of spreadsheet working will have become apparent and can be ameliorated when working on the study data.

While the spreadsheet can easily meet the needs of even quite large studies without advanced computing skills, more sophisticated data checking, manipulation and statistical analyses may be afforded by the use of database programs and statistical packages. In a larger study it is likely that at least one member of the team will contribute specialized skills to enable the use of these more sophisticated computer packages.

A final general point worth making about handling data on a computer is that modern computer programs are ergonomically designed and flexible. As a result they generally work in a natural or intuitive fashion most of the time. Having said that, the very nature of the computer is that it is extremely stupid; any behaviour that conveys a semblance of intelligence is a result of a programmer anticipating what the user wants (a good example of this is the word processor that corrects the author's typing mistakes. Each time I type the letters 'hte' it replaces them with the letters 'the'). When it comes to data handling or manipulation you will find that the programmer may have been less kind. Although the spreadsheet program will happily allow you to type in the data in rows or columns and most of the functions will happily work with data in either format, you may find that some functions are easier to use if you place your data in a particular format. If spreadsheet data are going to be exported into another statistics program it is important to check at an early stage if the statistics program expects the data in a particular format as it may well not be flexible. The 'take home' message from this paragraph is that you should be prepared to adapt to the way the computer works in order to make life a bit easier, rather than expect the computer (or its programmer) to work on data laid out in a form that you think is more logical.

13.3   Planning the management of data

The steps in data management are listed in Table 13.1.

The key tasks during the design phase are to define and name each variable, set up the database and test the database. During data col-

Table 13.1   Steps in data management.

1	Define the variables
2	Set up the database and data dictionary
3	Pre-study testing of data management
4	Data entry and error checking
5	Document data changes
6	Database backups
7	Create dataset for analysis
8	Final archiving

lection the main tasks are the entry of data, error checking and backing up the data.

13.4   Definition or coding of variables

13.4.1   *Variable names*

Each variable needs to be given a short name that is used within the program. Although many programs can handle names that are up to 250 characters long, and can include almost any character, it is best to keep names relatively short. Fewer than eight characters is the safest limitation (a few older programs have this limitation so it may be worth checking before assigning names) but 12 or fewer is normally safe. It is best to restrict names to letters and numbers and not use spaces within the name, an underscore character ('_') is safe to use where a space might be desirable. Try to avoid using the same characters for more than the first few letters for multiple variables (e.g. haematology_hb, haematology_mchc, haematology_pcv) as some programs may allow longer variable names to be imported by truncating them (by deleting the last few letters). It clearly helps to give them mnemonic names and a record will be kept in the data dictionary (see below) describing exactly what data are stored in the variable.

It is often helpful to be consistent in how variable names are assigned by deciding on a rough rule of using up to the first six letters of the long name followed by an underscore and then a number for the sequence if this is a repeated measure

Table 13.2   Examples of variables that might be used in a veterinary study.

Question	Variable name	Type	Format	Permitted values	Logic check
A	Spey	Integer	Yes No Missing	$=1$ $=0$ $=-1$	Value should be 1, 0 or −1
B	Agespey	Integer	2–144 missing	$=2-144$ $=-1$	Value should be −1 to 144 when A = 1
C	Incont	Integer	Yes No Don't know Missing	$=1$ $=0$ $=2$ $=-1$	Value should be −1 to 2

(e.g. creati_1, creati_2, creati_3, for three serum creatinine levels measured on three occasions).

13.4.2   The data dictionary

Within the database (whether it is stored in a spreadsheet or as a database) the data from each set of results are stored as a series of records. Each record consists of fields containing the values for each of the variables. The data dictionary contains a definition of each variable. This is a working document that defines the database. It should contain the following information about each variable or field:

- the short name or code for the variable
- a long descriptive name of what the variable is
- the type of the variable (e.g. integer, floating point number, logical, text, etc.)
- if it is mandatory (e.g. the animal's identity number)
- should it be unique (e.g. there should only be one record for each animal)
- any limits on the value it contains (e.g. an age in years should be greater than 0 and less than 18)
- consistency rules (e.g. the age at neutering should only be included if the animal has been neutered).

The long name for the variable is an essential piece of information because no matter how obvious the mnemonic used for the short name there is always a time when we can't remember which variable is which. Similarly, abbreviations that make sense to one member of the team may not be as obvious to another investigator.

All computer data management software allows for the storage of text and numbers in different formats. There isn't scope in this chapter to go into much specific advice to cover all eventualities. When using a spreadsheet to store data, and especially when this data is going to be analysed within the spreadsheet, integer coded values should be used for limited response questions such as the sex of an animal (i.e. entire male, entire female, neutered male and neutered female). Even when the natural inclination would be to enter these values as text or coded text (e.g. M, F, NM, NF), a better approach is to establish a coding system (e.g. M = 1, F = 2, NM = 3, NF = 4). In database programs that allow the user to enter text items from a list the database actually encodes the data in this way in its internal workings. Using integers like this makes the statistical analysis much simpler and will ensure that if the data have to be exported to a statistics package there will be no need for complex conversions. Although this method has the disadvantage of not being particularly transparent (although more sophisticated spreadsheet users will be able to create a more ergonomic user interface), it also ensures that data are entered consistently. If investigators are entering free text they might decide to enter the sex as 'speyed', 'spayed', 'castrated', etc., which will cause considerable problems down the line. The important point to bear in mind is that inconsistent data entry will ruin any attempt to analyse the data and must be avoided at all costs.

At this stage it is probably worth thinking about dealing with missing data. The key variable in the data will probably be the animal or sample's identity number or code. This field will be mandatory and probably unique; missing data in this field will be unacceptable. Other data may quite reasonably be omitted. However, it is possible that this data might be missing rather than not applicable. For this reason it is often better to have a code that represents explicitly the fact that an attempt was made to obtain the data but it was not available (e.g. 'not known' = 5). This will avoid further attempts to contact the owner or client for this information.

The remaining information in the data dictionary facilitates the data-checking process. Essentially it consists of rules that restrict the data and can be used to identify gross errors either at the data entry stage or before analysis. In database programs there are usually fairly straightforward options that can be chosen during the database setup to implement these rules and flag up errors during data entry. Error checking when using spreadsheets requires more sophisticated techniques but is still possible.

13.4.3 Setting up the database and testing

Having created a first version of the data dictionary the next step is to consider how the data are to be analysed. If this is being done by a third party, or a specialist member of the research team, they should be consulted to obtain details of their requirements for the format of the final analysis data set. They may be happy to receive a copy of the spreadsheet or database file, or they may stipulate an exported data format with records in either rows or columns. Their scrutiny of the data dictionary will also provide valuable input and is likely to uncover potential problems that the investigator may not have spotted.

At this stage the database or spreadsheet can be set up, including any data entry forms (both paper and electronic) that may be required. Having completed this, a dummy run using fabricated data should be completed to cover every step of the data entry, editing and analysis. The fabricated data need only consist of a small number of records but the whole process should be followed, including the statistical testing of the main hypothesis. While this may seem somewhat laborious, it provides the only realistic way of ensuring there are no fundamental problems with the data-handling and analysis system. In studies with a pilot phase the data generated from this can be used.

At the end of this stage a final version of the data dictionary and data entry forms will have been produced. This provides a good milestone that indicates that it is now safe to proceed with the main study.

13.4.4 Data entry and error checking

Data generated from the study should be recorded directly onto forms specifically designed for the study. There are considerable advantages in avoiding direct entry into computerized forms even though there may be some transcription errors when the data is eventually entered into the study database. Paper forms provide a permanent record of the raw study data, they are highly portable, they require no special skills and when well designed they impose few restrictions on how they are completed. There may be problems with legibility, particularly if there are corrections. It is best to encourage the clear crossing out of erroneous data, rewriting of the correct data, and initialling and dating the correction. For this reason it is often helpful to leave a reasonable amount of white space within entry boxes or between entry boxes.

Data should be transferred into the computer as soon as is practicable. This should enable errors or inconsistencies to be identified while the author or owner/client is still available to read their own handwriting or recall events. The layout of the computer screen should reflect the layout of the paper form. Drop-down lists can be used to assist data entry when they are available, and checking that the data entered is within the expected range will also help to trap errors at this stage. Typical problems with keyboard entry are confusing the letter 'o' with the digit '0', and the letters 'I' or 'l' with the digit '1'. Another problem is either omitting a decimal point or putting it in the wrong place.

While these more obvious errors can be flagged using a sophisticated user interface, other transcription errors may not be easily identified. Manual checking of a sample of paper forms against the data stored on the computer will give some indication of the scale of the problem. If the quality of the data is of the utmost importance it can be double-entered and the two entries compared to each other. Any inconsistent pairs can then be compared to the paper original to determine the correct data. In small studies each form entered can be double-checked after entry, either by the person who entered the data or, preferably, a different person.

13.4.5   Changes to the data

The integrity of the study can be affected by a failure to keep a record of any changes to the data. However legitimate the reason for editing (e.g. misrecorded data that are subsequently corrected), clear evidence that the study's results have been tampered with in the absence of any justification will be seen as suspicious. Whenever there are any changes to the study data some record of who performed the edits, what data was affected and why the change was made should be recorded.

13.4.6   Backing up the data and archiving

There appears to be a direct correlation between the time since the last backup and the likelihood of a computer failure. Regular backups are absolutely essential. A formal process of maintaining at least three backup copies of the study files housed in different locations should be diligently followed. Thefts of laptops, hard disc failures and simple human error are regularly responsible for the loss of, in some cases, many years of work. This can be avoided by keeping multiple copies.

The simple act of copying is not a guarantee of avoiding the loss of data. There have been some notable examples of a rigorous backup regime being followed but because the corrupt files were copied over the top of previous versions and the corruption was not noticed until some weeks after the event, all the backup copies were corrupt as well. This was understandable in the days when backup media (e.g. discs and tapes) were relatively expensive but the use of write-once optical discs (CD-ROMs and DVD-ROMs) should avoid this at a very low cost. The biggest risk occurs with mislabelled or poorly labelled disks.

Once the study has been completed it is highly desirable to create a study archive. Because computer programs and storage media may become obsolete, a paper copy should also be kept, which is not likely to be affected by the rapid advance in technology. The original computer files in their original formats should also be archived together with a universal export format (i.e. as ASCII text files), which should ensure that the data continue to be accessible even when the original program or hardware cannot be used.

13.4.7   Creating the analysis data set

The study database should be subject to a final quality check and editing cycle before the analysis phase. It should be frozen at this stage and established as the final copy. From this file one or more analysis files will be produced. The data may need to be exported to another package and if there are incompatibilities between the study database formats and the statistics package there may need to be changes to variable names, etc. This will only occur if there has been inadequate planning. If it does happen an appendix should be added to the data dictionary to clearly document the mapping of the new variable names to the old variable names.

Because studies rarely examine a single simple hypothesis it is likely that there will be numerous data subsets that are required to perform different analyses. In some statistical packages these are handled within the program. When using a spreadsheet it is often easiest to create multiple files or sheets containing different subsets of the data. Consistent naming conventions and careful organization of the different files will help avoid confusion and time wasted working on the wrong data set. It may be many months after performing the analysis that questions arise from the reviewing of the results when a manuscript is submitted for publication. The maintenance of a record of the file names and the analyses performed in the study log will ensure that any additional analysis required can be completed with a minimum of extra effort.

13.5 Further reading

Dohoo I, Martin W, Stryhn H (2003) A structured approach to data analysis. In: *Veterinary Epidemiologic Research*, AVC Inc., Charlottestown, Prince Edward Island, pp 581–90.

Kumar R (2005) *Processing Data*, 2nd edn, Sage Publications Ltd, London, pp 219–46.

Hulley SB, Cummings SR, Browner WS, Grady DG, Newman TB (2007) Data management. In: *Designing Clinical Research*, 3rd edn, Lippincott Williams and Wilkins, Philadelphia, pp 257–69.

13.6 MCQs

1 *When should development and testing of the data management system be performed?*

(a) Before the study begins.
(b) After data have been collected.
(c) During the statistical analysis.
(d) When writing the paper reporting the results.
(e) After the results have been published.

2 *What is the best format to store a variable recording body temperature measured in °C?*

(a) As a text variable.
(b) As an integer variable.
(c) As a floating point variable.
(d) As a categorical variable.
(e) As a logical variable.

3 *What is the disadvantage of collecting both 'age' and 'date of birth' of subjects?*

(a) Collecting both pieces of information creates redundancy (i.e. wastes storage space).
(b) Age may be recorded in days, months or years and so will be inconsistently recorded.
(c) Age can be calculated from date of birth.
(d) Date of birth can be calculated from age.
(e) As they are effectively the same datum recording it twice introduces the potential for conflicting values.

4 *How frequently should data be backed up?*

(a) Daily.
(b) Weekly.
(c) Monthly.
(d) Every 2 weeks.
(e) At an interval that minimizes the work required to re-enter the data.

5 *How many backup copies should be kept?*

(a) 1
(b) 2
(c) 3
(d) 4
(e) 5

6 *What is a data dictionary?*

(a) A dictionary of technical terms used by the trial.
(b) A definition of statistical jargon.
(c) A formal description of each variable name, format, permissible values, consistency checks, etc.

(d) An internal file in a relational database.
(e) The data management rules.

7 *Which of the following is a technique to identify potential data entry errors?*

(a) Double entry of data.
(b) Manual checking of a proportion of data.
(c) Formal training and certification of data entry staff.
(d) Examination of the distribution of values within a data field.
(e) Setting up the data entry system to flag anomalous data (e.g. text when a number is expected).

8 *How long should the raw data from a study be kept for?*

(a) Until the data have been analysed.
(b) Until the study report has been written.
(c) Until the study report has been published in a journal.
(d) For 1 year after the publication of the report.
(e) For several years (or as long as is practicable) after publication of the report.

9 *Which of the following types of software can be used to process study data?*

(a) A word processor.
(b) Presentation software.
(c) A spreadsheet program.
(d) A database package.
(e) Specialist statistical software.

10 *What course of action should be taken when an error in a data file is detected?*

(a) Analyse the data as it is and ignore the error.
(b) Correct the data and proceed to analysis.
(c) Correct the data, record the correction in the data log and proceed to analysis.
(d) Discard the data file and re-enter the data from scratch, as there may be other errors.
(e) Analyse the data omitting the erroneous data.

13.7 MCQ answers

1. (a); 2. (c); 3. (e); 4. (e); 5. (c); 6. (c); 7. All the answers can be used to reduce or identify errors in data entry; 8. (e); 9. (c), (d) and (e); 10. (c)

14

WRITING A RESEARCH PROTOCOL AND APPLYING FOR FUNDING

Objectives

After reading this chapter readers should:

- be aware of sources for clinical research funding
- understand the structure(s) of a grant proposal
- understand the grant review process
- understand the grant awarding/monitoring process
- be able to write grant proposals.

Good clinical research starts with a simple focused research question. Writing the research protocol forces the investigator to consider all the practical aspects of performing the research to a high standard. It helps to organize, clarify and define all elements of the study. Even when additional funding is not required the protocol is an essential element needed to perform the study.

A research proposal is an instrument used to justify the project. It is normally prepared for the consideration of a funding body and contains the background to the research question, the protocol, a budget and other administrative details as required by the funding agency. This chapter focuses on the structure of the proposal and introduces some of the common conventions.

14.1　Writing a proposal

As with every other area of enterprise the likelihood of success is dependent on good planning and hard work. Not only does the value of the proposed research have to be communicated but also the quality of the methodology and the ability of the investigator(s) to complete the research successfully.

14.1.1　*Where will the proposal be submitted?*

Each grant-awarding body has its own remit for providing support and its own application procedure. Details of these should be obtained at an early stage. This will determine the submission dates and levels of funding available, and contain the specific details they require, usually in the form of guidance notes for applicants.

Most funding bodies will not consider applications that are being considered by other agencies and may also ask if this application (or a similar one) has been submitted before. This means that the best chance of securing funding will be the first attempt. For this reason it is important to select the most appropriate source of funding first. Look for positive and negative factors. If 80% of the projects a body funded during the previous funding round were similar to your application, this may make them more reluctant to fund more of the same this time round. On the other hand, if the funding body has announced that they want to make research in your area of interest a priority then this may confirm them as the best choice.

14.1.2　*Who is going to do the research?*

It is generally the larger studies that require funding. These proposals require input from several team members. The team may be small, consisting of the investigator and a mentor (or supervisor), or it may require input from collaborators, a statistician, an accounting administrator and support staff. The team leader is often referred to in documentation as the principal investigator (PI). Some funding bodies require the PI to be a full-time employee of a research institute or university, and if the team leader is in veterinary practice it may be necessary to collaborate with someone who is prepared to supervise the project and act as PI. For inexperienced practice-based team leaders it is essential to be able to demonstrate that there is sufficient experience within the team. In any event inexperienced researchers will benefit enormously from the input from a more experienced mentor.

14.1.3　*Follow the instructions of the funding body*

Almost all funding bodies provide clear instructions that cover the work that they will fund and the instructions on obtaining that funding. There is absolutely no point in ignoring these. Inevitably there are more requests for money than there are funds available. Funding bodies will therefore be looking for legitimate reasons to decline an application and one of the most obvious reasons is that the instructions weren't followed even if the project itself is eminently fundable. It may be useful to create a checklist of criteria for funding, of tasks to be performed and information that is required, to avoid missing a minor item that might otherwise be overlooked.

14.1.4 Organization and scheduling

Distributing the tasks and establishing a timetable are important elements of project management. It is probably worth establishing the dates of project meetings to review progress and agree on the final proposal. The timetable will be dictated by the submission date(s) of the funding body. Where university accounting bodies are involved it is important to consult them at an early stage to establish how much time they will require to approve the budget. Similarly, departmental approval procedures may need to be included in the timetable.

Produce an outline of the project proposal. This will provide a starting point for writing the proposal and organizing the tasks to be done. The writing is rarely performed in a linear process from page 1 of the application form to the end. Parallel working on a literature review and the protocol will often provide a more creative process as the search for information on methodology turns up more information on the background to the study and vice versa.

14.1.5 Research the funding body

Find out what research projects the funding body has funded in the past. This information is usually readily available on their website. The veterinary world is relatively small and it is likely that one or more members of the team will know some of the previously successful applicants.

Even when there are no personal contacts it is worth asking for advice from a successful applicant. If possible obtain a copy of their application. This will give a clear indication of the level of detail and language conventions that have been successful in the past. Previously funded investigators are often used as grant reviewers and although this is a confidential process people are often happy to talk in general terms about the types of flaws that should be avoided. There is often some benefit from speaking to an administrator at the funding body even if only to reconfirm any detail that is not clear from the instructions received.

The membership of the final grant-awarding panel of the funding body may also be published and a friendly member of the panel may be willing to provide informal advice on the suitability of an application for funding. A word of caution should be sounded here. Some potential applicants might be tempted to believe that recruiting a panel member as a collaborator may give an application some advantage. Sadly the opposite may be the case, as a panel member with an involvement in a project is likely to be excluded from any decision on an application in which they have an interest.

While most applicants are diligent in the preparation they put into the technical aspects of their proposal they don't put as much effort into their research of the funding process and yet this research may make the difference between success and failure.

14.1.6 Write, review and revise

Proposal writing is an iterative process and the commonest problem with most grant proposals results from the failure to allow enough time for it (usually due to trying to get a grant application written a short time before the grant deadline).

The proposal will be subjected to a grant review process similar to that used by scientific journals for papers that are submitted to it. A 'peer', an experienced veterinary clinical researcher working in the field, will be asked to critique the application. Applicants should ensure that the proposal has been subjected to the same level of scrutiny as a journal article before it is sent off. Look at it critically and try to anticipate any potential flaws or weaknesses. Alter the proposal if necessary and at the very least make it clear that these areas have been considered carefully, different options have been considered and include contingency plans for any likely problems.

Apart from the intellectual rigour of the internal reviewing of the document, care should be taken to remove any typographical errors and inconsistent nomenclature, use correct naming conventions and ensure the aesthetic appearance of the proposal. These factors may not affect the quality of the science but their absence suggests an inability to pay attention to detail or a tendency towards carelessness, which will not inspire confidence in the proposal.

14.1.7   Pilot data

The presentation of a proposal from an inexperienced investigator or a proposal for work in an entirely novel area is often enormously strengthened by the inclusion of pilot data.

The collection of this data demonstrates unequivocally the fundamental feasibility of the technical aspects of the project and shows that the investigators are likely to be competent to perform the work proposed. Pilot data may establish the hypothesis is reasonable in the face of expert opinion that has the weight of experience (or at least seniority) even if there is no other evidence to support the opinion. A final advantage of pilot data is that it is likely to strengthen the confidence in any sample size calculations that are presented.

14.2   The elements of a proposal

Each funding body has its own form design and application procedure. Larger funding bodies now require applications to be made using internet-based systems. All these formats contain similar elements. This section examines the different elements in the proposal formats normally required from all funders of veterinary clinical research. No one funding body lays out their proposal form in the exact order and in the same detail as is described below but they all follow a similar pattern.

14.2.1   The first section

Inevitably this consists of some basic information about the proposal, not least of which are the names, addresses and contact details of the applicants. There are two important elements that bear a little consideration: the project title and an abstract of the project proposal.

The title may be asked for in two forms: a short title to provide a less unwieldy handle for the project to be referred to for administrative purposes and a longer, more informative title for more widespread use. The title should be descriptive and concise. It provides a lasting reminder of the content and design of the study. A well-worded title manages to encapsulate these elements, achieving brevity by avoiding unnecessary phrases such as 'A clinical trial to determine the ...'. The choice of title is important and it may influence the decision made by grant-awarding panels.

Together with the title, the abstract gives readers their first impression of the proposal. Reversing any negative impressions gained at this stage will be an uphill struggle. The abstract is a concise summary of the protocol which should state the research question, include the study design and methodology, and conclude with a statement indicating the importance or relevance of the potential findings of the research. It is highly likely that the abstract will be restricted in length. It is nearly always one of the last elements of the proposal that is written. By this stage 'proposal fatigue' may well have set in. Resist the temptation not to give the abstract the same degree of attention as the rest of the proposal. It should be reviewed and edited just as with any other section. It may well be the only part of the proposal that is read by some reviewers and it will certainly be referred to as an aid to memory when the panel discusses the application. It should be able to indicate the intentions of the study, its strengths and its value in it own right.

A second, non-technical abstract may be requested. The main use for this is to convey the content of the proposal to a lay audience in publicity should the grant be awarded. Remember that there may be a lay person on the awarding panel, particularly with some of the smaller grant-awarding bodies, and so time spent on this is not wasted.

14.2.2 Administrative information

A variety of administrative information will be required which may include budgetary details, staff details, resources available, need for a Home Office Licence (UK only), ethical approval, management plans, institutional approval, etc. Of these the most important items are the budget and its justification.

It is likely that both a summary of the budget (early in the form) and a detailed budget, including justifications, are required. For budgets including staff costs there will undoubtedly be requirements from the university or research institute administration for consultation and approval of pay scales, increments and overheads.

The budgeting process is best started at an early stage partly because it has an influence on the overall feasibility of the proposal but also because it may require the collation of information from a variety of sources and may take some time. A budget hastily put together at the last minute is unlikely to impress a reviewer and may lead to considerable under-estimating of the true cost of the project. Within reason, try to think of all the possible expenses. The application form will lay out different categories of costs and within these sections items like staff costs

(where applicable), travel, animals, equipment and consumables will be listed. Each individual item should be identified, costed and justified.

The budget is not expected to be set in stone, and minor variations in expenditure will not require permission from the funding body. It is sensible to estimate a maximum number of assays, tests, etc. to allow for working-up procedures or repeated tests. Major changes in the protocol may have significant effects on expenditure and investigators should certainly consult the funding body before any significant non-budgeted funds are committed in variance to the original agreed budget.

An indication of the amount of time to be devoted to the project by various members of the team may be requested. Where key members of the team are only contributing a small proportion of their time (say 5%) to the project and are listed as being involved in a number of other research projects, there may be some doubt as to their commitment to the proposal under consideration. Reviewers will also look at the overall experience levels of the team and it may be quite appropriate for a senior member of the team to contribute primarily in a supervisory role.

The application form will undoubtedly require some form of biographical details for the named investigators. These will include details of recent publications and research funding received. Where there are significant contributions from collaborators, signed letters of agreement will also be required.

Where existing facilities from the host institution provide an important contribution to the resources required to complete the study these should be listed. They may take the form of access to expensive shared equipment such as laboratory equipment or the use of animal-handling facilities. There may be costs associated with these both in the processing of individual subjects or animals and in the requirement for a contribution towards the annual maintenance costs of running the resource.

14.2.3　The aims, objectives and importance of the work

The first section of the scientific part of the proposal is similar to the introduction of a scientific paper. The exact format will vary from funding body to funding body. It is normally not necessary to provide an extensive literature review but it is sensible to refer to any work that has directly influenced decisions or ideas that are presented in the proposal.

The specific aims should be statements of the research question that describe in concrete terms the desired outcome. Each aim should be succinctly described in one or two sentences. Where there are multiple aims these should be set out in order of importance or chronologically (reflecting the sequence in which they will be achieved).

This early section may be entitled 'Aims and objectives' without a clear indication about what is meant by an 'aim' and what is meant by an 'objective'. Looking at previous successful proposals may help to indicate what is acceptable. It may help to consider the aims as the questions being asked and the objectives as the significant milestones that allow these questions to be answered. In recent years greater thought has been put into the instructions and the formats of application forms and they are reasonably explicit about what is expected.

The application instructions will indicate where the importance of the proposed work is to be described. This may be in a separate section or be included in the aims and objectives. Although the proposal is likely to be reviewed by someone familiar with the field of proposed research, it is possible that not all members of the decision panel will have this familiarity. For this reason the value and importance of obtaining the anticipated results should be comprehensible to someone who is not an expert in the field. Sufficient information should be given to make it clear what this particular study will accomplish and why it is important. In specific terms, how will the findings from this study advance our understanding or change clinical veterinary practice?

14.2.4　Details about the methods to be used in the study

This section will subsequently be expanded into the operations manual for carrying out the study. It will receive considerable scrutiny from the reviewers and is where a significant number of applications fail. Sometimes the instructions will indicate the structure that should be used and may ask for a schematic diagram indicating milestones and timing. Even if these are not asked for they are useful to clarify the overall structure of the plan and indicate that attention has been paid to identifying critical points and the management of the project. The specific components of the methodology that are likely to be used are covered elsewhere in this book. The recruitment of animals, the measurements to be taken, the pilot phase, data management, quality control and the plans of analysis should all be described. Detailed descriptions of laboratory techniques may not be required. When established techniques are being used suitable references can be cited, otherwise detailed descriptions can be provided in an appendix if these are allowed.

Some application forms will have a separate section for statistical analysis, which should include the plan for analysis. This can be laid out in a logical sequence starting with the variables to be collected and the approach to be used to test associations. This will lead on to the subject of sample size, which should begin with a statement of the null hypotheses to be tested and the justification for the statistical test to be used and then the sample size and power estimates with the selected alpha error, beta error and effect size. Reviewers often attach a lot of importance to the statistics section and when it appears credible and error free it suggests that considerable thought has been put into how the research question will ultimately be answered. There is considerable value in obtaining the assistance of a statistician to help write or review this section.

14.2.5 References

The proposal should be adequately referenced. Where statements of fact that are not supported by results or data are provided in the body of the proposal they should be referenced. The quality of the references used sends a message about the applicant's familiarity with the field. The references should be comprehensive and balanced, reflecting the current state of knowledge. There is no need for an exhaustive indiscriminate list of citations covering the entire history of research in this area. Be careful to read the papers that are referred to and not just rely on abstracts or copying the citations made by others. Sloppy mistakes in the inappropriate use of references, misinterpretations of their results and inaccurate citations will serve to irritate reviewers, who may well be the authors of some of the papers cited.

14.3 What are the characteristics of a good proposal?

A successful proposal is one that addresses a good, focused research question and clearly demonstrates the technical quality of the study designed to answer that question. To some extent these aspects are self-evident. However, even if the question and the technical quality are of the first order the proposal may fail due to poor writing and presentation. A vague discursive narrative will cause the reviewer to lose interest when it becomes difficult to follow the reasoning of the author. On the other hand, a clearly laid out and worded proposal is easy to read and understand.

Consider the poor reviewer, faced with a pile of lengthy proposals. Concisely written, well-organized proposals that use headings, sub-headings and white space between paragraphs or sections will take far less time to read and understand. Use of diagrams, tables and lists may also help to speed up the reviewing process.

Avoid the use of hyperbole or exaggeration in addressing the importance of the study. Reviewers are naturally sceptical and are more likely to be won over by reasoned argument and logic. Be realistic about any limitations in the project and be willing to identify any inescapable weaknesses in the study design. These will require a certain degree of risk assessment or cost-benefit consideration to minimize their importance. However, there is also a risk in excessive humility; there is no merit in drawing the reviewer's attention to a multitude of minor problems that might otherwise be overlooked. The proposal should aim to reassure the reviewer that the investigator(s) has anticipated the potential problems and has a realistic and intelligent approach to dealing with them.

In an ideal world the applicant should leave enough time before the submission date to have someone with excellent language skills read the proposal to check for clarity, and spelling and grammatical errors. This person need not have any expertise in the research described but may provide a final stylistic polish to the document.

14.4 What happens once the proposal has been sent?

The next step naturally depends on the mechanisms employed by the funding body. Inevitably there is a delay, which may be up to 9 months, before a decision is communicated to the applicants. There should be an indication of the likely decision time in the instructions to applicants.

Organizations deploying a large amount of money will undoubtedly use a formal review process, which may occur in three stages. Firstly, the administrative staff will check applications for adherence to the instructions that were provided. The proposals will then be sent out for review to between one and three reviewers with expertise in the field in which the proposed study is based. One or more of these reviewers may be on the decision panel, which then meets to rank the applications and allocate funds. This panel is likely to consider the applications in two passes. During the first pass any seriously flawed proposals will be culled from the list to leave a list of proposals that are considered worthy of funding. From this list the proposals will be ranked in order of merit. The most meritorious proposals will be allocated funds and the less meritorious may be allocated funds if there are funds remaining after the better proposals have been funded. The feedback to the applicant is likely to be 'not considered suitable for funding', 'a good proposal but unfortunately insufficient funds were available in this round' or 'we are pleased to tell you that your proposal has been selected for funding'.

The amount of feedback provided to failed applicants is highly variable and is often not provided unless specifically requested. As considerable time and effort goes into both writing a proposal and its review this can be extremely frustrating. Applicants should be encouraged to ask for feedback, particularly early in their clinical research careers. It may be possible to obtain some informal feedback by asking a senior colleague to contact a 'friend' on the decision panel. It may even be worth swallowing one's pride and taking a failed proposal to colleagues for their opinion (it is even better to do this before submitting the application). Failure rates are generally very high and everyone who regularly submits proposals for funding has their own tale of woe concerning particularly bitter failures.

Most failures are explicable and often arise from either overambitious plans or allowing insufficient time to write the proposal. The main reason that success breeds more success is that experienced successful clinical researchers represent a safer investment. The grant-awarding bodies are normally the custodians of public money or charitable funds and they feel that their responsibility is to be judicious rather than risk-taking in the way they administer their resources.

The best advice that can be given to failed applicants is to be honest and self-critical about their proposals before re-applying for funding. Consider starting with relatively modest projects with lower costs and also consider working with a collaborator with an established track record. There is only one certainty when it comes to grant applications and that is if you don't write one, you definitely won't get one.

14.5   Sources of funding

There are a variety of sources of funding available for veterinary clinical research. The remit of the different funding bodies and the amounts available will vary over time. For investigators working in universities or research institutes, access to information about sources of funds is normally not a problem. For veterinarians working in practice, recruiting a collaborator or mentor who is an established researcher will clearly help. Certain funding bodies, particularly those distributing large amounts of public funds, will require the grant to be held by a research institute or university department, and for the principal investigator be a full-time employee.

A list of organizations that fund veterinary research in the UK is given below. The list is not exhaustive and before making any application readers should approach the organization for current details of the funds available and the grant-awarding procedure.

RCVS Trust
http://www.rcvs.org.uk/
Belgravia House, 62-64 Horseferry Road, London SW1P 2AF
Tel: 020 7202 0714

BSAVA Petsavers Grants
http://www.petsavers.org.uk/home/resources/grants/

British Small Animal Veterinary Association, Woodrow House, 1 Telford Way, Quedgeley, Gloucestershire, GL2 2AB
Tel: 01452 726700

The Horse Trust (formerly the Home of Rest for Horses)
http://www.horsetrust.org.uk/
Speen, Princes Risborough, HP27 0PP
Tel: 01494 488464

The Horserace Betting Levy Board
http://www.hblb.org.uk/
52 Grosvenor Gardens, London SW1W 0AU
Tel: 020 7333 0043

The Wellcome Trust
http://www.wellcome.ac.uk/
Gibbs Building, 215 Euston Road, London NW1 2BE, UK
Tel: 020 7611 8888

Biotechnology and Biological Sciences Research Council (BBSRC)
http://www.bbsrc.ac.uk/
Polaris House, North Star Avenue, Swindon, SN2 1UH
Tel: 01793 413200

14.6   Further reading

Hulley SB, Cummings SR, Browner WS, Grady DG, Newman TB (2007) Writing and funding a research proposal. In: *Designing Clinical Research*, 3rd edn, Lippincott Williams and Wilkins, Philadelphia, pp 301–316.

Kumar R (2005) Writing a research proposal. In: *Research Methodology*, 2nd edn, Sage Publications Ltd, London, pp 187–206.

15

WRITING AND REVIEWING SCIENTIFIC PAPERS

Objectives

After reading this chapter readers should:
- understand the formal structure of a scientific paper
- understand the process of writing a paper
- appreciate the conventions of style and presentation
- be able to critically appraise a scientific paper.

15.1   Introduction

Communication is essential to get your scientific work into the outside world. This may take the form of talks, posters or publications. Publication of your work is important if your work is to be recognized. This chapter will focus on the writing of a scientific paper for publication in a peer-reviewed journal. Also included in this chapter is information about how to review a scientific paper. These are two sides of the same coin and are complementary in understanding what makes a well-written paper.

15.2   Writing scientific papers

15.2.1   Style

As with any form of writing, style and accuracy are important. Clear, simple, accurate composition with good grammar and accurate spelling is vital to ensure that your reader can understand your work. There are also some conventions about scientific writing that you must know. For example, when numbers are used with a unit of measurement (e.g. 2 kg) or with a noun (e.g. Group 4) numerals are used. When used independently as numbers, e.g. 10 rabbits, numbers less than 10 are written as words, e.g. four, and numbers 10 or above are written as numbers, e.g. 23 goats. Some of the more important rules of scientific writing are described in the following sections.

15.2.2   Referencing published work

When information derived from other published work is used in a paper it should be referenced. This means that it is cited by either a number (used sequentially through the paper) or the author's (or authors') name and year. Names and dates are indicative of when and who performed the cited work whereas numbers do not interrupt the flow of the text. For each journal you have to follow the style given in the instructions for authors.

The citation should appear in the reference list at the end of the paper. The reference list gives details of where the source information can be found. The reference usually contains the year of publication, the journal it was published in, and the volume and the page numbers. For each journal you have to follow the style given in the instructions for authors.

The citation can be made as either part of a sentence or at the end of a sentence.

Name and date system

Experimental evidence indicates dogs have four legs (Jones 1996)

Jones (1996) observed that dogs have four legs

Reference list

Jones, J.J. (1996) Observations on the number of legs dogs have, Journal of Leg Counting, 4, 1–4

Number system

Experimental evidence indicates dogs have four legs.[1]

Jones observed that dogs have four legs.[1]

Reference list

1.   Jones, J.J. (1996) Observations on the number of legs dogs have, Journal of Leg Counting, 4, 1–4

Most journals instruct authors to use the abbreviation 'et al.' or use the words 'and others' (Latin *et allii* means 'and others') when references are cited with more than two authors. For example, if a paper by Jones, Smith and Harris (1999) is cited,

Jones et al. (1999) or Jones and others (1999) would be the citation in the text.

If more than one publication of an author or the same group of authors published in the same year are cited in the paper using the name and date system, these have to be distinguished. This is achieved by adding a letter to the year, e.g. 1988a, 1988b.

If several publications relate to the same statement these are cited in either chronological or alphabetical order, for example in alphabetical order (Ashley 2005, Barker 1982, Carter 1992, Davis 1988) or, more usually, in chronological order (Barker 1982, Davis 1988, Carter 1992, Ashley 2005).

Books are not primary literature and some editors and reviewers may reject them when cited. However, if statements can only be supported by book references they can be cited in the same way as described for primary publications and most journal instructions for authors provide the format required for the reference list.

If statements are supported by unpublished works the acknowledgement of the source of the information is required. The citation is in the form (J.J. Jones, personal communication). There is no entry in the reference list. Some journals will reject unpublished citations.

15.3   The structure of a scientific paper

A well-written scientific paper must fulfil two objectives. Firstly, it must clearly and completely describe the procedures that were followed and the results that were obtained in such a way that the study could be repeated using the paper as a source of instructions. Secondly, it must place these results in perspective by relating them to the existing state of knowledge and interpreting their significance for future study.

In order to be able to write or appraise a scientific paper an understanding of the formal structure

Table 15.1

The research process	The scientific paper
1. The scientific question	Introduction
2. What is known and not known	Introduction
3. Formulate problem	Introduction
4. Hypothesis	Introduction
5. Project plan	Materials and Methods
6. Experiment and collate data	Materials and Methods
7. Analyse results	Results
8. Interpretations and conclusions	Discussion
9. New knowledge	Discussion
10. New questions	Discussion

is necessary. Scientific papers usually include the following major sections or major headings:

- Title
- Authorship
- Abstract
- Introduction
- Materials and methods
- Results
- Discussion
- Acknowledgements
- Literature cited

Many journals have a type of scientific paper entitled Short Communication, which has the same format as other papers but with a reduced word limit and restricted headings.

To understand the organization of a scientific paper it is worth examining the major steps in the research process and how these relate to the sections in a scientific paper (Table 15.1).

The sections of a scientific paper reflect the organization and content of the research process. Each section of a scientific paper will now be described.

15.3.1   *Title and authorship*

Title

This describes the contents of the paper. A good title is straightforward and uses keywords that researchers in a particular field will recognize. The title should be to the point, but descriptive, letting the reader know exactly what the paper is about.

Authorship

The list of authors should only contain the individuals who made a substantial intellectual contribution to the research. This may include the people who were involved in composing the conceptual idea, obtaining funding, designing and supervising the experiments and writing the paper. Technical assistance should be included in the acknowledgements. The first author has usually made the largest contribution but may not necessarily be the person who wrote the paper. Ensure all the authors have read the final manuscript before submission and that their current addresses, qualifications and titles are correct.

There has in recent years been a trend to longer and longer list of authors on papers. To some extent this is merely a reflection of the increasing need for collaboration in technology based research, but it also reflects the fact that paper authorship is an easily measured index of research performance much loved by bureaucrats. In general it is a greater sin to omit the name of someone who has substantially contributed to a study from the list of authors than to include someone who might not deserve to be listed. In one of the authors' experiences (MAH) the omission of an author on one of his papers caused considerable unhappiness; it costs very little to acknowledge an important contribution in this way and it is often much appreciated.

15.3.2   Abstract and keywords

Abstract

The abstract should provide the context or background for the study and state the study's purposes, basic procedures (study design, subjects, observational and analytical methods), main findings (giving specific effect sizes and their statistical significance) and principal conclusions. It should emphasize new and important aspects of the study or observations.

The objective, materials and methods, and the results are usually written in the past tense while the discussion and the conclusions are in the present tense.

Keywords

Some journals request keywords, usually between 5 and 10. These are important and should be chosen with care. Database search functions use keyword indexes to identify relevant papers.

15.3.3   Introduction

This must outline the scientific purpose(s) or objective(s) for the research performed and give the reader sufficient background to understand the rest of the paper. Only background that is pertinent to the experiment should be presented. All statements of fact should be supported by an appropriate citation, which is indicated in the text and included in the list of references. The introduction sets the stage for the rest of the paper and should highlight gaps in current knowledge. The introduction should end with a clear statement of the purpose of the study. This may be phrased as a hypothesis to be tested or as a question to be answered. A good introduction will answer several questions, including the following:

- Why was this study performed?
- What knowledge already exists about this subject? The introduction should present a review of the literature, showing the historical development of an idea and including the confirmations, conflicts and gaps in existing knowledge.
- What is the specific purpose of the study? The specific hypotheses and experimental design pertinent to investigating the topic should be described.

Use the present tense to write the motivation and hypothesis but use the past tense for the literature review and the objective.

15.3.4   *Materials and methods*

This section answers all the basic questions about how the study was done so that another scientist could repeat your study. It requires considerable discipline and effort to be accurate and comprehensive in the descriptions of what was done while at the same time avoiding excessive detail or verbosity. The author should assume that the reader has a similar level of education but is not necessarily familiar with the techniques or technology employed. It is appropriate to cite other papers that describe the methodology used; however, it is important to note any variations or modifications that may have been used in your study. It is extremely frustrating as a researcher, when attempting to follow the methods used described in a paper, only to realize as you embark on the work that insufficient detail has been provided for you to replicate the methodology. This section should answer the questions 'Where and when was the study done?' and 'How was the study done?'. There should be sufficient detail to allow the reader to decide whether the data that are presented in the results section are likely to be accurate. Any statistical methods used to analyse the data should also be described here, citing a source for the use of the statistical tests, perhaps a statistics book or program.

The overall design and protocol

This section should contain information regarding the overall design and protocol, the subjects used, treatments and interventions and the statistical analysis. This should include the definitions of the study groups (placebo, control and treatment groups), the procedures undertaken or treatments given and whether the investigator collecting the data was blinded to eliminate bias, that is denied access to knowledge of which treatment group the data were being collected from. The power of the study should be stated if possible. The power of a study is the probability of detecting an effect in the treatment versus control group if a difference actually exists. It must also specify the size of the difference. For example, a paper describing a clinical trial with a new mastitis treatment may contain the following statement: 'The study had a power of 80% to detect a difference of 10 000 cells per ml in milk between the treatment and control groups'. Typical power probabilities are 80% or greater.

The subjects

These should be clearly defined. In a study of a particular disease, the inclusion criteria, including the formal case definition (the basis on which the diagnosis was made), should be provided. Subjects vary according to sex, age and breed. Ideally, in a well-designed study, the subjects should be selected so that the treatment groups are comparable. Matching the groups will limit the effects of sex, breed and age on the results of the study.

Treatments and interventions

It is necessary to define the reagents used, doses, concentrations and the routes of administration, in order for the reader to clearly understand the procedures undertaken.

Statistical analysis

Most statistical methods are well known and simply need to be stated (e.g. analysis of variance, Student's *t* test and Fisher's exact test). Complex and unusual analyses should be described and referenced in detail. Methods for computing standard statistics such as the mean, standard error, standard deviation, confidence intervals and percentiles do not need to be described or referenced.

The past tense should be used for the materials and methods. References to genus and species should be accurate. Drugs and chemicals should be referred to by their chemical names with the product name and manufacturer provided. The correct technical name of equipment used and the manufacturer should be given.

15.3.5 Results

The results section should summarize the data from the experiments without discussing their implications. This section should concentrate on general trends and differences and not on trivial details. Results should clearly describe what was found and not require the reader to interpret data from figures and tables. The data should be organized into tables and figures. Generally, results include only summarized data and observations obtained in the study. The inclusion of raw data is not necessarily required but authors may choose to make this data available either on request to the author or by providing an internet location from which it may be obtained.

Figures and tables should include a legend so as to be self-explanatory, that is the reader should be able to understand what they describe or contain without having to refer to the main body of the paper. The same data should not be presented in both tabular and graphical form unless there is a compelling need. Figures are useful to illustrate relationships and tables are best when specific numbers are important. Follow the journal instructions regarding the construction and labelling of figures and tables. When using figures ensure there is consistency with the number of decimal places and accuracy described, and that the accuracy implied by the number of digits provided is appropriate for the measurement accuracy (e.g. providing body temperatures to three decimal digits is ridiculous). Make headings meaningful and include the units. Remember, figures may be reduced in size for publication so be careful when constructing complex diagrams. Select the best type of figure to illustrate your results. These may be pie charts, bar charts, line graphs or scatter diagrams. Avoid unnecessary ornament such as a three-dimensional effect on bar charts. With line graphs do not place too

many lines on one graph and use the scales to best effect. Do not use dotted lines. Use colour only when it is essential, as you may be charged for this.

Statements about the significance of differences examined by statistical tests should contain a precise indication of the test used and the probability level chosen. The results should clearly state the power of the experiment, the statistical significance and the confidence intervals of the data. The mean and standard error are usually expressed in the form mean $\pm$ SE. The terms 'significant' for $P \leq 0.05$, 'highly significant' for $P \leq 0.01$ and 'very highly significant' for $P \leq 0.001$ are used by some but not all journals.

The past tense should be used to refer to the results.

15.3.6 Discussion

Conclusions or interpretations and the implications of the results are discussed in this section. The conclusion portion restates the primary goal of the research, the hypothesis and whether the data and results collected support or reject that hypothesis. It is important to remember that any statement of fact should be supported either by the results reported in the study or other published results, which should be cited appropriately. The findings should be related to the present state of knowledge and future needs for research. Make sure this is genuinely interpretive, not just a restatement of the introduction or results sections. This section should identify sources of error and any inadequacies of the research. This is important because it is the author's opportunity to pre-empt the likely criticism of the reviewers (see section 15.6.1). Nobody expects every clinical study to be performed flawlessly and it increases the confidence of the reviewer to see the limitations of the study and its results put into context by a well-reasoned discussion. This also helps to avoid misleading the clinicians who might use the evidence generated by the study. The goal of the discussion, and indeed the whole paper, is to enable the reader to make an informed decision as to how they use the knowledge generated.

In the discussion the present tense is used when interpreting the results and referring to the works of others.

15.3.7   Statement of interests

A number of clinical journals now require all authors to make statements about potential conflicting interests. Within the veterinary clinical research field pet food manufacturers and drug companies may provide funding for research or for posts, which should be acknowledged here. What is required is usually explicit in the instructions to authors provided by the journal.

15.3.8   Acknowledgments and literature cited

Acknowledgements

These are optional, depending on the study. Give credit to those who helped in your research through advice, work, permission, technical advice and monetary support.

Literature cited

This contains only those items specifically referred to within the text. Authors should read the cited literature carefully to ensure that the statements made about that paper are supported by the contents of that paper. While it might be tempting just to rely on the citations used in another author's published paper, this should be avoided and you may well highlight your ignorance by repeating another person's error (which is likely to spotted by a good reviewer). Try to avoid excessive lists of citations describing a single phenomenon or well-accepted fact. It is quite acceptable to cite a review paper or to indicate that the citation is just one representative of many similar observations.

15.4   Selecting a journal

Journals vary in the subjects that they accept. Some are highly specialized whilst others are more generalized. Each journal will indicate their scope on their websites and within the journal. It is important that you select the journal you wish to submit your article to carefully to avoid a rejection by the editor on the basis of an inappropriate topic for the journal. It is also worth giving careful consideration to your target readership. Is it purely for the research community or is it for clinical veterinarians as well? The citation index of a journal is an indirect measure of the impact that the journal has on scientific research in general. Journals therefore have a hierarchy of importance. This index has to be interpreted with care as papers in low-citation journals may still have importance in a specific context. Once you have decided which journal to send the paper to (and remember you only send it to one journal) it is vital that your paper conforms to the instructions for authors for that journal.

15.5   Instructions to authors

All journals provide instructions to authors, which can be found in back issues of the journal or on the journal's website. It is crucial that these are read carefully and adhered to. Journals vary in the length of the article permitted, their method of referencing of authors, whether coloured figures will need to be paid for and the format of the submitted manuscript, amongst other things. They also indicate the number of copies of the article that should be sent, the form in which the manuscript is required (paper and/or electronic) and where to send it. Although not always stated, clarity of writing and correct grammar are expected. Ensure that you have checked the manuscript thoroughly for spelling errors, format and coherence.

The instructions provided by the journal *The Veterinary Record* are reproduced in Figure 15.1 as an illustration.

Contributions in the form of original research papers, review articles, clinical case histories, short communications and letters on all aspects of veterinary medicine and surgery are invited. All except letters are refereed. Submissions are accepted on the understanding that they have not been published elsewhere and that they are subject to editorial revision. All material published is the copyright of The Veterinary Record.

FORMAT

Manuscripts should be typed, double-line spaced, on one side of the paper only and with wide margins. A covering letter and three copies of the manuscript should be submitted together with three sets of any illustrations. All abbreviations should be spelt out in full the first time they are used in the text. Medicines should be referred to by the generic name, followed by the proprietary name and manufacturer in brackets when first mentioned; e.g., fenbendazole (Panacur; Hoechst).

PAPERS

Papers should include a title of not more than 15 words, the names, qualifications and addresses of each author, and a summary of not more than 200 words. They should be set out in the following sections: summary, introduction, materials and methods, results, discussion, acknowledgements and references. Clinical papers or case reports should follow a similar overall arrangement, modified appropriately. The text should be as concise as possible; the whole length should not exceed 4000 words (that is, about four to five pages of *The Veterinary Record*). Please also supply five keywords to accompany the paper.

SHORT COMMUNICATIONS

Preliminary accounts of work and short clinical reports for publication as short communications should follow a similar format to papers but should exclude a summary and separate subheadings. The title should be no more than 10 words in length, the text should not exceed 750 words and only one or two figures and/or tables should be included. Please also supply five keywords to accompany the short communication.

LETTERS

Letters on all topics related to the science, practice and politics of veterinary medicine and surgery will be considered for publication. They should be typed in double-line spacing on one side of the paper only. The length should not exceed 400 words and the editor reserves the right to shorten letters for publication. They must be signed by the author(s). References should be quoted only when absolutely necessary. Illustrations and tables suitable for reproduction will occasionally be allowed.

TABLES and ILLUSTRATIONS

Tables should be kept to a minimum and presented separately from the text. The legend should clearly explain what data the table is presenting without the need to refer back to the text. Tables should not duplicate information presented in figures. Line figures and photographs will normally be reproduced at column width (76 mm). The author's name, title of the paper and number of the figure should be pencilled lightly on the back of each illustration. Colour or black and white transparencies and

Figure 15.1 The instructions to authors provided by the journal *The Veterinary Record*. (Copyright 2005. The Veterinary Record, London, UK)

prints are acceptable. Where transparencies are submitted, they should be accompanied by a set of prints. Prints should be clear and sharp. X-rays should be submitted as good quality prints. Histograms should be presented in a simple, two-dimensional format, with no background grid; tones should be avoided.

REFERENCES

In the text references should be cited as follows: Smith (1995) described.../...recorded earlier (Brown and Jones 1994, Smith and others 1997). Lists of references should be given in date order in the text but alphabetically in the reference list.

In the reference list all authors' names and initials should be given followed by the date, title of the paper, full title of the journal, volume number and full page range, e.g.: SMITH, A. B., JONES, C. D. & BROWN, E. F. (1995) How to list your references. *Veterinary Record* 151, 71-76

Book references should include the chapter title if appropriate, the full title of the book, the edition, the editors, the town of publication, publisher and page numbers of material referred to, e.g.: SMITH, A. B.,JONES, C. D. & BROWN, E. F. (1993) How to list your references. In *Getting It Right*. 3rd edn. Eds S. Adams, J. Alexander. London, Society of Reference Publishers. pp 23-37

MEASUREMENTS

Measurements should be expressed in the metric system or in SI units. Temperatures should be given in °C. Centrifugation speeds should be given in g.

ETHICS

Papers may be rejected on ethical grounds if the severity of the experimental procedure does not appear to be justified by the value of the work presented.

Figure 15.1 (*cont.*).

15.6 The peer review process

The reviewing process may be a very unhappy experience for the clinical researcher. While the euphoria of having completed and written up the study rapidly dissipates, the fear of rejection looms.

For inexperienced researchers or authors, it is highly advisable to precede the formal reviewing process with an informal review. If you already have a supervisor or mentor they will be prepared to read the paper and provide feedback. They may also be able to suggest a suitably qualified person unfamiliar with your study who might provide a useful objective view. At the very least you should ask friendly colleagues to provide some feedback. Meticulous checking of the language used (particularly if you are not writing in your native tongue), data presented, the references, etc. will avoid giving the reviewer unnecessary (and unwelcome) work which might not endear them to your paper.

If you have avoided any major methodological flaws (which if you've read this book you should have), written the paper with due consideration to the instructions to authors (and the guidance in this chapter), and the editor considers your paper of interest and relevance to the journal's readership then the paper should ultimately be accepted. It is highly unlikely that the reviewers will not find some faults or suggest some improvements but after you have made some modifications it should be accepted for publication.

Following the receipt of the reviewers' reports the editor will write to you. The paper may be rejected outright and reasons are usually given. It may be accepted without modification or it may be accepted with certain specified major or minor modifications.

Once the paper has been submitted the editor or sub-editor will acknowledge the receipt of the article and indicate it has been sent to reviewers for comment. It is usual to send the article to two reviewers who have experience in the subject of your paper. It is instructive to be aware of what the reviewers are looking for and what they are being asked to do. Below are the instructions provided by the *Equine Veterinary Journal* to its reviewers.

Instructions to reviewers

Refereeing involves critically appraising the positive and negative aspects of a paper. Referees are likely to ask the following generic questions when reviewing a paper (Malmfors et al. 2004):

Basic questions

- Has the author conveyed his or her message clearly?
- Is the aim, hypothesis or problem clear?
- Are the facts presented clearly?
- Are the references given when needed?
- Do the facts support the conclusions?
- Are the structure and layout correct and appropriate?
- Is anything missing or superfluous?

Detailed questions

- Does the title of the paper accurately reflect the content?
- Is the abstract complete and does it stand alone?
- Is the subject material relevant to the journal?
- Is the experimental design appropriate for the hypothesis being tested?

- Are the methods appropriate and fully described and referenced?
- Is the statistical analysis correct?
- Are the results presented properly?
- Is the material duplicated in text, tables or figures?
- Does the author interpret the results correctly?
- Does the author describe non-significant differences as though they were significant?
- Could alternative interpretations or conclusions be drawn from these results?
- Does the paper make a significant contribution to the literature?

A referee's checklist is often provided by the journal. The checklist used by the *Equine Veterinary Journal* is shown in Fig. 15.2.

15.6.1 Editors' and referees' reports

If modifications are requested, once they are completed it is best to send a covering letter to the editor to indicate how you have addressed each issue raised by the reviewers.

If the paper has been rejected it is useful to reflect carefully on the reviewers' comments before deciding whether to submit the article to a different and perhaps more appropriate journal. Remember, the peer review process is not infallible and if you feel that the reviewers' comments are unjust write to the editor with your reasoned arguments. The editor may send the manuscript out to other reviewers if your arguments are valid.

15.7 Copyright and proofs

Once accepted, the paper will be prepared for publication. The technical editor may have further questions about your paper regarding an incomplete reference or other errors and ambiguities. The editor will also send you a form regarding the copyright of the paper and the publication of your paper. You will be asked to

```
EQUINE VETERINARY JOURNAL
REFEREE'S CHECKLIST


Title:

Author(s):

Date:

        _____



1) Is the question being asked worthwhile and will it make a valuable addition to
knowledge?                                                        Yes/No*

2) Does the experimental design adequately test the hypothesis or answer the
question?                                                         Yes/No*

3) Are the methods appropriate?                                   Yes/No*

4) Are the data presented accurately and clearly?                 Yes/No*

5) Are the data interpreted correctly and are the conclusions reached
appropriate?                                                      Yes/No*

6) Does the title indicate the nature and scope of the paper?     Yes/No*

7) Are the references appropriately and accurately cited?         Yes/No*

8) Are there adequate references to other publications?           Yes/No*

9) Are the tables and figures:
        (a) necessary?                                            Yes/No*
        (b) clear and labelled adequately?                        Yes/No*
        (c) provided with suitable titles?                        Yes/No*
10) Are you satisfied that there are no factual errors or inconsistencies?  Yes/No*
    _____


If you answer NO to any of the above, please give further details on the Referee's
Report to Author
```

Figure 15.2 The referee's checklist used by the *Equine Veterinary Journal.*

sign a copyright agreement with the publisher of the journal before the paper is published.

You will also be sent author proofs if you are the designated corresponding author. This is the copy of your paper that will appear in the journal and it is your last chance to check and change it. The proofs may be either electronic (usually pdf files) or hard copy. Usually only technical or formatting errors should be identified and corrected, although minor modifications may be allowed. It is best to work on a copy of the proof. Every aspect of the paper, including spelling and data, should be checked with the utmost care. The proof marks should be entered into the proof, with the corrections neatly written in the margins. Proof marks are annotations that have specific meanings that can be used to highlight in the text the correction that is required. Request a list from the journal if they want you to use them. Alternatively identify the errors in the text and clearly explain in the margin the correction that is required. Return the corrected proof as quickly as possible to avoid any delay in publication.

15.8   Reference

Malmfors B, Galsworthy P, Grossman M (2004) *Reviewing Papers and Presentations in Writing and Presenting Scientific Papers*, Nottingham University Press, Nottingham, pp141–2.

15.9   Further reading

Bowers D, House A, Owens D (2001) *Understanding Clinical Papers*, Wiley, New York.
Crombie IK (1996) *The Pocket Guide to Critical Appraisal*, BMJ Publishing Group, London.
Day RA (1998) *How to Write and Publish a Scientific Paper*, 5th edn, Cambridge University Press, Cambridge.
Greenhalgh T (2001) *How to Read a Paper*, BMJ Publishing Group.
Malmfors B, Galsworthy P, Grossman M (2004) *Writing and Presenting Scientific Papers*, Nottingham University Press, Nottingham.
Mason I (1995) Writing and publishing a paper in a veterinary journal. *J Small Animal Prac* **36**: 214–20.

Matthews JR, Bowen J, Matthews RW (1996) *Successful Scientific Writing*, Cambridge University Press, Cambridge.

15.10   MCQs

In which section of a scientific paper are you likely to find the following:

1   *The formulation of the problem*

(a)   The abstract or summary
(b)   Introduction
(c)   Materials and methods
(d)   Results
(e)   Discussion

2   *Analysis of results*

(a)   The abstract or summary
(b)   Introduction
(c)   Materials and methods
(d)   Results
(e)   Discussion

3   *Experimental details*

(a)   The abstract or summary
(b)   Introduction
(c)   Materials and methods
(d)   Results
(e)   Discussion

4   *New scientific questions*

(a)   The abstract or summary
(b)   Introduction
(c)   Materials and methods
(d)   Results
(e)   Discussion

5   *New knowledge*

(a)   The abstract or summary
(b)   Introduction
(c)   Materials and methods
(d)   Results
(e)   Discussion

6   *Hypothesis*

(a)   The abstract or summary
(b)   Introduction

(c)   Materials and methods
(d)   Results
(e)   Discussion

7   *Interpretations and conclusions*

(a)   The abstract or summary
(b)   Introduction
(c)   Materials and methods
(d)   Results
(e)   Discussion

8   *The scientific question*

(a)   The abstract or summary
(b)   Introduction
(c)   Materials and methods
(d)   Results
(e)   Discussion

9   *Project plan*

(a)   The abstract or summary
(b)   Introduction
(c)   Materials and methods
(d)   Results
(e)   Discussion

10   *What is known and not known*

(a)   The abstract or summary
(b)   Introduction
(c)   Materials and methods
(d)   Results
(e)   Discussion

15.11   MCQ answers

1. (b); 2. (d); 3. (c); 4. (e); 5. (e); 6. (b); 7. (e); 8. (b); 9. (c); 10. (b)

16

ETHICAL AND LEGAL CONSIDERATIONS

Objectives

After reading this chapter readers should:

- know the appropriate legislation, particularly the Animals (Scientific Procedures) Act 1986
- be able to recognize if a study is likely to require a licence
- be aware of the GCP guidelines that may be relevant to a study
- understand some of the ethical issues that may impinge on a study
- understand the requirements for informed consent by clients.

There are a number of ethical and legal issues that impinge on veterinary clinical research. Inevitably most of the legal aspects will be specific to the country in which the research is being performed while the ethical issues are more universal. This book was authored in the UK and readers from other jurisdictions should seek advice from their local authorities and veterinary registration bodies for specific advice.

16.1   Ethical considerations

A comprehensive account of all the many ethical issues that surround veterinary clinical research is beyond the scope of this textbook. The main risk to veterinarians involved in clinical research is that they lose sight of their duty of care to their individual patients in their pursuit of research results to help the larger population. Each study must be judged on its own merits and each patient should be treated as an individual.

16.2   Ethical principles

The consideration and application of ethical principles represents an entire academic discipline in its own right. There are three main principles that should be considered: respect to subjects, beneficence and justice.

16.2.1   Respect for subjects and people

This requires investigators to obtain informed consent from the clients or owners of the animals that are involved in studies, consider the welfare of the animals involved and maintain confidentiality. It is important to remember that the animals and their owners are not passive sources of data, but individuals whose rights and welfare must be respected. Veterinary researchers should always uphold their duties and responsibilities as a veterinarian as their first priority, and pursue their research aims as a second priority.

16.2.2   Beneficence

The principle of beneficence requires that the research design be scientifically sound and that any risks be acceptable in relation to the likely benefits. Apart from any risks to patients it is also important to consider any psychological effects on the owners. Many owners see their pets as members of the family and may react strongly to apparent discomfort or suffering in their animals. It may be possible to reduce risks to subjects by introducing exclusion criteria that identify animals more likely to suffer adverse responses to treatment. All aspects of the study design that increase the likelihood of detecting a useful outcome, and all aspects that seek to decrease any pain, suffering, discomfort or lasting harm, increase the beneficence of the research.

16.2.3   Justice

This principle may seem more appropriate in clinical research performed on people. It states that the benefits and burdens of research be distributed fairly. In other words that vulnerable populations aren't used as experimental subjects or fail to benefit from the research due to unequal distribution of health care. Good practice-based veterinary research should ensure that the population most likely to benefit from the study actually provides the test population.

16.3   Ethical review

The best strategy to avoid ethical problems is to go through a process of ethical review during the planning stage. It is far better to use inclusion criteria that eliminate any foreseeable clinical problems that might occur than to face the dilemma of an unplanned withdrawal as a result of animal suffering or owner/client unhappiness.

Questions that should be considered during the ethical review process are:

- Have the risks to participants been minimized?
- Are the risks reasonable in relation to the anticipated benefits and the importance of the knowledge that might be expected to result?
- Is the selection of participants equitable?
- Will informed consent be obtained from the owners or clients of subjects?
- Will the integrity of data and any confidentiality be maintained?

16.3.1 Ethical review boards

All veterinary schools and research institutes will (or should) have an ethical review board or panel whose remit is to scrutinize research proposals for ethical difficulties. If an investigator is working outside such an organization they may find that the ethical review board of a local institute or veterinary school will be willing to review the clinical research proposal and provide feedback. At the very least the investigator should ask colleagues to examine the work that is proposed for possible ethical issues.

16.4 Informed consent

A key issue in veterinary clinical research is obtaining the informed consent of the clients or owners of the animals being used as subjects in the study. This is a complex issue and goes far beyond obtaining a signature on a consent form.

Most of us imagine that when we consult a medical practitioner and agree to treatment that we have gone through a process that involved our giving informed consent to the treatment that we receive. Interestingly, a study of medical prac-

titioners in the USA looking at the decisions made about patients' treatment during consultations carried out by Braddock et al. (1999) concluded that fewer than 1 in 10 decisions met the criteria of an informed decision (i.e. included discussion of the nature of the decision and asking the patient to voice a preference). If this happens in the highly litigious culture pervading North America it is likely that the situation is at least as bad elsewhere.

16.5 Criteria for informed decision making

There are seven criteria that should be met to ensure that the person providing consent can truly be said to have given informed consent.

Firstly, clients need to know that they actually have a role in the decision-making process and that their views or opinions will influence the decision that is being made. The essential point that they need to know is that if they do not want to participate in the research study they aren't compelled to do so, and that their refusal will not be detrimental to the treatment their animal receives.

Clients need to understand the nature of the decision being made. They need to know that this is not an irrevocable decision and that they may withdraw from the trial should they become unhappy with the situation once the trial has begun.

They need to know what the alternatives are. In a normal consultation we would normally explain which diagnostic options or alternative treatments are being considered.

They should understand what the risks and benefits are. This is particularly important. The communication and understanding of risk are notoriously difficult. Individual personalities have very different perceptions of risk. There may be few hard data on which to base a risk estimate. The investigator will not wish to frighten a client into declining to participate but on the other hand there is the need to ensure that the client understands that there is a finite and tangible risk.

Leading on from this is the need for the client to appreciate that there is a degree of uncertainty. Evidence from previous studies may lead to a relatively high confidence that a new treatment has a lower incidence of adverse reactions but pure chance may have produced more favourable results and masked the real level of side effects.

Clients must have an opportunity to express any failure to understand. Clients come to the clinic with a wide range of educational backgrounds and may be intimidated by their surroundings and the 'white coats'. It is important that the investigator or member of staff obtaining consent knows enough about the study to be able to answer any questions that arise and it is even more important that the client knows that any questions they may have will be answered. Do not rush the process or give the impression of impatience.

There should be an exploration of client preference. At the end of the consent process the clients must be given a clear opportunity to decline to be involved.

16.6   Practical guidelines on obtaining consent and avoiding problems

The first point that has already been made is that the ethics of a proposed study should be explicitly considered at the planning stage, preferably taking advantage of a formal external review by an ethics committee or panel. The results of this review should be documented and included as an appendix to the protocol or proposal. A copy of a letter of approval of an ethical review panel is often a useful document to provide to collaborators and the clients or owners of subjects.

The second important area is communication with clients or owners of the animals, both when obtaining consent and during the conduct of the study. The two key documents that are likely to be used are the consent form itself and a document containing information and instructions for the clients and owners. Both these documents should be written with care to ensure that all the information is accurate and correct, but they should also be written in language that a lay person might reasonably be able to understand. Jargon and technical language should be avoided where possible. This doesn't mean that the documents shouldn't contain a full description of the study but some background information may be necessary in order for someone without a veterinary education to understand what will happen. Proof reading by non-veterinary qualified individuals should help to get the wording and language pitched at the right level.

The main client information and instructions may end up being quite a large booklet. Many of us are daunted by long technical documents but we all tend to read at least the first page. Use this page wisely and ensure that the key information is contained on this page; if appropriate use the first page as a summary of the whole document. Give clear instructions on the taking of any samples or any measurements that you are expecting the clients/owners to take. It is better to over-document what is required with step-wise simplistic instructions and diagrams than to leave it up to the clients/owners to guess what was intended. What may be obvious to the investigator may be utterly opaque to a non-veterinarian. When it is important to identify animals that have adverse effects following an intervention or where there is a need to identify any deterioration in the patient's condition, try to give practical information to help clients/owners understand exactly what to look for.

Make sure that there are good channels for communication and that these are spelt out in the client/owner information document. For example, there may be an instruction to telephone the practice emergency line if concerned, but this will be of little use if the reception staff or agency that provides emergency out-of-hours cover know little about the study. A standard operating procedure (SOP) on handling client/owner concerns should be written and implemented. This may necessitate some training for reception or out-of-hours staff or may require a separate emergency number for the study.

Another area that should be explicitly and unequivocally stated in the client/owner documentation is that of costs. Most studies undertake to cover the costs of any procedures carried out as part of the study and the treatment of adverse events that might reasonably be the result of an intervention carried out during the study. Some clients may be under the impression that this means they will receive free veterinary treatment throughout the study. To avoid this impression it may be necessary to state that the occurrence of an unrelated disease or an accident (e.g. a road traffic accident) will result in the withdrawal of the animal from the study and the subsequent costs of treatment will be the responsibility of the client.

The consent process should be described in another SOP. The important components of this form are a concise description of what will happen to the animal if the owner/client provides their consent, any significant risks and a statement that the form should not be signed if the client/owner has not had an opportunity to ask any questions or does not understand any part of the form. It may also be wise to require a veterinarian to countersign the form to say that they have provided an opportunity for the signatory to ask for clarification or to answer any questions.

16.7   Other ethical issues

16.7.1   *Randomized controlled trials*

The principal ethical dilemma in performing a randomized clinical trial is in the use of two or more treatments that might not be believed to be equally effective. While this is not surprising as it is normally the reason for performing the study,

investigators have to make an ethical decision on the unequal risks faced by subjects receiving a less effective treatment. This is most starkly highlighted by the use of a placebo group. The ethical basis for assigning treatment by randomization is the judgement that both arms of the protocol are in equipoise (i.e. are balanced). This is important when the risks of a failure in treatment are high, as would be the case in, for example, a systemic bacterial infection. In other cases, e.g. mild skin disease or late stage terminal cancer, the imbalance between treatment arms is less likely to affect the final outcome detrimentally. Judgements about the comparison groups to be used should be based on the existing evidence on the efficacy of treatments together with the clinical context.

16.7.2   *Research on previously collected specimens and data*

This topic has not presented any problems in veterinary clinical research in the recent past, but veterinary researchers should be aware of the potential pitfalls. The retention of cadavers or pathological material and their subsequent use in research should not be performed without explicit permission from owners. The use of tissues such as blood left over from normal clinical sampling or additional sections from biopsy specimens is unlikely to be resented, and permission for their use is unlikely to be refused. Simple additions to the consent forms and client advice information will ensure that problems are avoided.

16.8   Data protection legislation and confidentiality

There are two aspects to be considered. Firstly, there is legislation (the Data Protection Act 1988 in the UK) that limits the storage and use of personal data and secondly there are the practical steps that should be taken to ensure confidentiality. Veterinarians have an obligation not to divulge information about clients or their animals to third parties without permission. All veterinary practices should be aware of the legislation regarding data protection and adhere to the principles laid down in the Act. Veterinary clinical research is a legitimate use for which personal data can be used as long as the clients are aware that this is one of the reasons why their information is stored. Once veterinary clinical data has been depersonalized (i.e. it can no longer be identified as belonging to a particular owner), there is rarely a problem with publishing that data. Replacing the identification of owners and animals at an early stage of data processing with identification numbers and ensuring that any document/file that reveals the link between numbers and identification is kept in a secure place and not distributed is advisable. All veterinary schools have a data protection officer who may be able to provide advice if researchers are unable to work on anonymous data or believe that there may be a problem.

16.9   The Animals (Scientific Procedures) Act 1986

There are two important pieces of legislation that may affect veterinary clinical research: the Veterinary Surgeons Act 1966 (VSA) and the Animals (Scientific Procedures) Act 1986 (A(SP)A).

In the UK it is illegal to hurt or harm animals under the Protection of Animals Act 1911 and subsequent amendments. A(SP)A establishes the legality of animal experiments providing they are carried out according to the stipulations contained in this Act. The Veterinary Surgeons Act establishes the right for suitably qualified and registered members of the Royal College of Veterinary Surgeons (RCVS) to perform acts of veterinary medicine and surgery. Although these veterinary procedures may cause some pain and suffering (e.g. administration of drugs, injections, surgery, etc,) they are intended to be beneficial to the animals under their care.

For the majority of veterinary clinical researchers the main aims are to avoid designing studies

that involve procedures that would fall under the provisions of A(SP)A and to restrict procedures to those that are recognized by the RCVS as acts of veterinary medicine or surgery. The question then arises as to what procedures fall under A(SP)A.

16.9.1   What is a regulated procedure under A(SP)A?

The A(SP)A protects all vertebrate species (and *Octopus vulgaris*) once they are capable of independent existence (e.g. early stage embryos may not be covered[1]). Regulated procedures include anything that causes pain, suffering, distress or lasting harm through either commission or omission. The threshold of regulation for pain, i.e. the point at which it is considered to be severe enough to fall under the Act, is generally held to be the equivalent of the skilled introduction of a hypodermic needle into or through the skin. Pain, suffering, distress and lasting harm are considered to be cumulative and so repeated application of a procedure causing lesser pain, or a series of procedures inducing a combination of minor pain, suffering, distress and/or lasting harm, might also be considered to be above the threshold for inclusion or regulation under the Act.

As has already been stated, recognized veterinary practices are exempt from A(SP)A, as are recognized agricultural practices, normal animal husbandry and humane killing by what is called a Schedule 1 method (this covers normal slaughter procedures).

---

[1] Embryos are covered by A(SP)A during the latter half of gestation or incubation for mammals, birds and reptiles. They are also covered if they are caused pain, suffering distress or lasting harm (PSDLH) prior to this, but then go onto full development and there is a chance that the regulated procedure applied at any stage of development may cause PSDLH later. Other species (e.g. amphibia, fish and octopus) are protected from the stage of independent feeding.

16.9.2 What constitutes a recognized veterinary procedure?

Before all members of the veterinary profession rub their hands with glee at the realization that acts of veterinary surgery are exempt from A(SP)A, they should first understand exactly what this means.

In an annexe to the *RCVS Guide to Professional Conduct* is the report of a working party to consider the interface between the VSA and A(SP)A. Veterinary clinical researchers should read this report carefully before conducting any clinical research. Some of the important points that are included in this report are given below:

'Acts of veterinary surgery (as referred to by A(SP)A) should be considered to be procedures and techniques performed on animals by veterinary surgeons in the course of their professional duties which ensure the health and welfare of animals committed to their care.'

'In all circumstances, the individual has to consider the primary purpose and whether he or she is acting in a professional capacity as a veterinary surgeon or as a research scientist. Although the procedures and techniques may be identical, analysis of the purpose for which they are applied should help the veterinary surgeon to determine if the intervention is of direct benefit to the animal or its immediate group and therefore recognised veterinary practice, or if the intervention is for an experimental or other scientific purpose and controlled by A(SP)A.'

'When conducting clinical investigations (without A(SP)A authorities) care must be taken to ensure that appropriate veterinary treatment and care is provided for all animals used in the study. The use of untreated "control" groups needs careful consideration, to ensure that no avoidable suffering results as a consequence of withholding treatments. The inclusion of placebo treated "control" groups will require A(SP)A authority if likely to cause pain, suffering, distress or lasting harm to the animal.'

'The use of any novel treatments must reasonably be expected to result in a similar or better outcome than that following conventional treatment. The veterinary surgeon must have some background knowledge of the treatment in order to make a professional judgement. When what is to be done has an experimental component, authority under A(SP)A may be necessary.'

'There are many examples where veterinary surgeons apply diagnostic tests and techniques to clinical cases that have already been developed for use in other species or human patients. Similarly, treatments used in human medicine may be introduced for use in animals where potential benefits might be expected for the individual animal or its immediate group, for veterinary public health or environmental protection. This is legitimate.'

The essence of these points is that anything that is done to an animal must be done for the direct benefit of the animal (or group of animals) and these animals must be under the care of the veterinarian concerned.

It is not acceptable to take a blood sample if the results from any test performed on that blood sample are not going to be used to assist in the diagnosis or treatment of that animal (or others in the immediate group).

It is not acceptable to use a placebo treatment if a disease has been diagnosed and not treating that disease will lead to pain, suffering or lasting harm. It is also not acceptable to give a placebo that would require an injection (e.g. the use of a saline injection as a control). Similarly, sham surgery is also not allowed without A(SP)A regulatory authority.

If these procedures are required as an essential part of the study design then applications will need to be made to the Home Office to have the study regulated under the A(SP)A.

16.9.3   How can research be performed without it coming under A(SP)A?

With a reasonable understanding of the provisions of the VSA and A(SP)A it is generally very easy for the vast majority of studies to avoid the need for A(SP)A licensing.

The first point to remember is that if the procedures are conventional veterinary treatments that would be considered acceptable veterinary diagnostic or therapeutic options for the treatment of the patient concerned there is no problem. If the study compares two conventional licensed therapeutics, in a randomized controlled trial, this does not fall under A(SP)A.

If a study wishes to compare two diagnostic tests, even if both tests cannot be performed on the same blood samples, as long as the information will be used to directly benefit the animal this should still fall under the VSA. The question the investigator should consider is whether or not the primary rationale for performing the tests is the benefit of the patient (which is acceptable) or the scientific study (which is not). Most veterinarians would argue that the results from two tests would provide a greater confidence in the result. Should the investigator wish to take six blood samples for six different tests then the authorities might be a little sceptical about the motivation.

Blood and other samples that are taken for legitimate diagnostic reasons can be used for research purposes. It is important that the primary reason for taking the sample is for the direct benefit of the patient and that the size of the sample is not excessive (i.e. not considerably greater than that which would normally be taken for the primary test).

The decision tree shown in Fig. 16.1 should help to provide some guidance as to whether the planned study may be subject to A(SP)A. Table 16.1 contains some illustrations that indicate how the RCVS and Home Office interpret A(SP)A and VSA in the context of clinical research. If the investigator is in any doubt they should seek guidance from their local Home Office inspector and the RCVS at the earliest possible stage.

16.9.4   An outline of the main relevant provisions of A(SP)A

Should veterinary clinical research have to be performed under the provisions of A(SP)A there are three main components to the licensing requirements: the project licence, personal licensing and the certificate of designation. Inspectors who are either veterinary surgeons or medics are appointed under A(SP)A to advise the Home Office on whether and on what terms these authorities might be granted. Performing studies that require licences should not be lightly undertaken and would normally be performed within a university or a research institute. This section provides a superficial description of the process and should not be regarded as definitive.

Project licences

The first requirement is to apply for a project licence. Careful scrutiny will be made of the proposed study to ensure that it has a permissible purpose under A(SP)A (e.g. the prevention, diagnosis or treatment of disease in animals) and that there is no alternative to using animals. The proposal will contain an account of the procedures to be carried out as well as the study design, including the justification and benefits. The Home Office inspector will weigh the likely adverse effects on the animals against the likely benefits. The inspector will have to be assured that all possible steps have been taken to minimize both the numbers of animals used and the suffering caused. The project licence will be held by a named individual who will have certain responsibilities of care to supervise the project and provide information to the Home

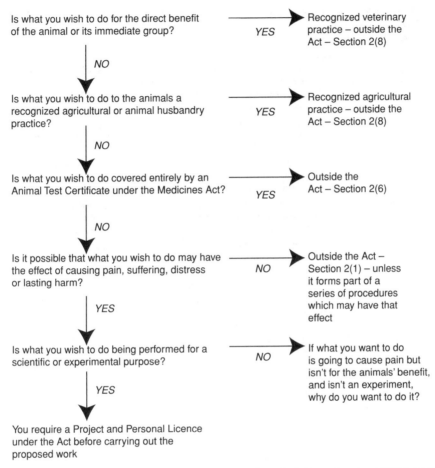

Figure 16.1 A flow chart to help establish if a proposed study falls under the A(SP)A 1986.

Office about the number of procedures that have been carried out.

Personal licences

To ensure the competence of anyone carrying out regulated procedures under A(SP)A there is a requirement for them to hold a personal licence. In order to obtain a personal licence individuals are required to be over a minimum age, hold suitable qualifications and have received specific personal licence training. While currently there is no charge for project licences, fees are associated with providing personal licence training and there is a fee for the personal licence itself.

Certificate of Designation

The place where the licensed research is performed has to be covered by a Certificate of Designation. Universities and research institutes normally hold these. There will be a certificate holder who accepts responsibility for the highest level of supervision. The certificate documentation includes the places where licensed research can be performed and specifies a named veterinary surgeon who has the overall responsibility for the health of animals kept for research purposes. Another named individual is the named animal care welfare officer, who is responsible for the general husbandry of animals covered by

Table 16.1 Examples of how terms used in the guidance provided by the Home Office and the Royal College of Veterinary Surgeons are interpreted in deciding if procedures are likely to fall under the Animal (Scientific Procedures) Act 1986.

Term	Examples
Direct benefit	• Taking blood samples from an animal, or animals, within a herd to assist in clinical management, e.g. diagnosis, metabolic profile • Taking a series of biopsies from an animal for diagnosis and monitoring the efficacy of treatment • Giving veterinary treatment to an experimental animal when treatment is for the animal's benefit • Use of drugs in ways other than described in product licence but for the direct benefit of animal concerned • Anaesthesia for a scientific purpose is regulated
Immediate group	• The herd or flock under the care of the veterinary surgeon • The pack of dogs or colony of cats under the care of the veterinary surgeon • The source animal in blood transfusion for use in clinical cases, but not on a larger commercial scale
Recognized practice	• Embryo transfer for expansion of colony, herd or flock for commercial reasons or to improve health status • Testing for halothane susceptibility in pigs • Restraint in commercial systems for husbandry purposes, e.g. stall-tied dairy cows • Laparoscopy for artificial insemination • Laparoscopy for observation of the gonads for sexing birds for non-experimental reasons • Removal of gonads or hormone administration for control of reproduction in non-experimental situations • Single housing of calves within the provisions of welfare codes
Not recognized practice	• Laparoscopy for observation of the ovaries for a scientific purpose • Feeding of diets at variance with normal practice, e.g. to induce the signs of dietary deficiency • Embryo transfer for scientific purposes • Harvesting blood or blood products on a larger commercial scale • Colostrum deprivation or early weaning for scientific purposes
No adverse effect	• Feeding of diets at variance with normal practice but which are not intended to result in deficiencies or excess of any dietary component • Restraint for up to 14 days where expression of normal behaviour is prevented
Adverse effect	• Any penetration of the integument, e.g. use of a needle • Any procedure requiring sedation or anaesthesia • Maintenance in restraint which significantly restricts expression of normal behaviour, for example close head restraint • Feeding of haematophagous insects
Scientific purposes	• Taking blood for blood products or laboratory use • Taking blood for teaching purposes • Taking biopsies to study the pathogenesis of a condition rather than to diagnose disease or monitor treatment in an animal • Inoculation of material into an animal for diagnosis of disease in another animal • Use of substances, drugs, etc. other than as described in product • Licence for research/development and not covered by an ATC

the certificate. The certificate holder is responsible for ensuring that codes of practice are maintained and followed, and that there is an ethical review process within the institution. There are provisions to enable clinical research to be performed in veterinary practices but the project licence must be held by someone working in an institution that holds a Certificate of Designation.

16.10 Veterinary Medicines Directorate Animal Test Certificates

It is possible to carry out certain clinical trials involving veterinary drugs under the authority of an Animal Test Certificate (ATC) issued by the Veterinary Medicines Directorate (VMD).

The majority of ATCs are issued to pharmaceutical companies to authorize the conduct of clinical field trials of products to confirm efficacy. These data then form part of the dossier of evidence for submission for a marketing authorization application. However, ATCs may also be issued for authorization of clinical research projects involving the unlicensed (off-label) use of an authorized veterinary medicine or for studies conducted for applications to extend or vary a current marketing authorization.

Although veterinarians may use unlicensed medicines in accordance with the provisions of the prescribing 'cascade', it should be noted that any trials conducted at the request of or on behalf of a third party require authorization by an ATC or under A(SP)A. Currently preclinical trials and early clinical trials can only be undertaken under the auspices of A(SP)A.

16.11 Good clinical practice

In spite of its rather generic sounding title, good clinical practice (GCP) is actually a set of quality assurance guidelines intended to give guidance on the best practice for running clinical trials (GCP was originally designed for human trials). Subsequently, an organization best referred to by the initials VICH (the International Cooperation on Harmonisation of Technical Requirements for Registration of Veterinary Medicinal Products!) developed a set of GCP standards that have been adopted in the USA, Japan and the EU. There are also related quality assurance programmes for laboratory work (good laboratory practice, GLP) and the manufacture and formulation of drugs (good manufacturing practice, GMP).

The main relevance of GCP to individual veterinary clinical researchers or practitioners is that should they become involved with clinical research in collaboration with pharmaceutical companies they may be asked to work to GCP standards. If this should occur they will be provided with the appropriate education and training but the following paragraphs provide a brief guide to the main elements of GCP.

The purpose of GCP is to establish guidance for the conduct of clinical studies that ensures the accuracy, integrity and correctness of the data produced. The use of pre-established systematic written procedures for the organization, conduct, data collection, documentation and verification of clinical studies is emphasized. The training, education and competence of those working on the study should be appropriate. Guidance is provided on what documentation is required and how it should be checked, logged and archived. The GCP guidelines indicate the roles and responsibilities of the investigator (the team leader of the group actually performing the work), the sponsor (normally a pharmaceutical company funding and benefiting from the study) and the monitor (an individual appointed by the sponsor whose responsibilities include quality auditing). Structure and contents for the main documents such as the study protocol, standard operating procedures and the final report are also provided in the GCP guidelines to a high level of detail.

Practical aspects of the implementation of GCP can be found in a book edited by Dent and Visanji

(2001) and a copy of the GCP guidelines can be obtained from the VICH website.

16.12   Reference

Braddock CH 3rd, Edwards KA, Hasenberg NM, Laidley TL, Levinson W (1999) Informed decision making in outpatient practice: time to get back to basics. *JAMA* Dec 22–29; **282**(24): 2313–20.

16.13   Further reading

Anon (2006) Annexe b. A(SP)A and VSA interface in *RCVS Guide to Professional Conduct*, RCVS, London (also available via the Internet http://www.rcvs.org.uk/).
Hulley SB, Cummings SR, Browner WS, Grady DG, Newman TB (2007) Addressing ethical issues. In: *Designing Clinical Research*, 3rd edn, Lippincott Williams and Wilkins, Philadelphia, pp 225–37.
Kumar R (2005) Considering ethical issues in data collection. In: *Research Methodology*, 2nd edn, Sage Publications Ltd, London, pp 209–16.
Pocock SJ (1983) Ethical issues. In: *Clinical Trials: A Practical Approach*, John Wiley and Sons, Chichester, pp 100–109.

16.14   MCQs

1 *Which of the following statements best describes the ethical concept of beneficence?*

(a)   That veterinary clinical research should not have adverse psychological effects on owners.
(b)   That research be scientifically sound and risks acceptable in relation to likely benefits.
(c)   That the test animals are taken from the population most likely to benefit from the results of the research.
(d)   That the views of owners are respected.
(e)   That the confidentiality of owners is respected.

2 *Which of the following is not a criterion required for informed consent?*

(a)   That clients know they have a role in the decision-making process.

(b)   That clients understand the nature of the decision being made.
(c)   That clients know what the alternatives are.
(d)   That clients know who to complain to if things go wrong.
(e)   That clients appreciate that there is a degree of uncertainty.

3 *Which of the following animals is not covered by the A(SP)A 1986 legislation?*

(a)   Locust.
(b)   Octopus.
(c)   Fish.
(d)   Cat.
(e)   Horse.

4 *Which of the following fall under A(SP)A legislation?*

(a)   Acts of veterinary medicine.
(b)   Recognized agricultural or animal husbandry practices.
(c)   Experiments that do not cause pain, suffering or distress.
(d)   A drug trial covered entirely by an Animal Test Certificate.
(e)   An experiment that does not cause pain but may cause lasting harm.

5 *Which of the following is not a recognized agricultural or animal husbandry practice?*

(a)   Removal of gonads for the control of reproduction for non-experimental reasons.
(b)   Laparoscopy for artificial insemination.
(c)   Sexing birds using laparoscopy as part of a research study.
(d)   Single housing of calves within the provision of welfare codes.
(e)   Testing of halothane susceptibility in pigs.

6 *Which of the following is not considered to be an adverse effect?*

(a)   Any penetration of the integument, e.g. use of a needle.
(b)   Any procedure requiring sedation or anaesthesia.
(c)   Keeping animals in restraints that significantly restrict expression of normal behaviour.

(d) Taking urine samples.
(e) Feeding of blood sucking insects.

7 *The VICH good clinical practice guidelines are:*

(a) a quality assurance scheme for veterinary practitioners
(b) a guide to professional conduct
(c) a quality assurance scheme for running clinical trials
(d) guidelines for continuing education
(e) a guide to veterinary laboratory practice.

8 *If an investigator has any concerns about the ethics of a study which sources of information could be helpful?*

(a) Colleagues.
(b) Professional bodies such as the RCVS.
(c) The Home Office.
(d) An ethical review board at a veterinary department.
(e) All of the above.

9 *What do the initials PSDLH stand for?*

(a) Plain-speaking dull little hermit.
(b) Pain, suffering, distress and little harm.
(c) Pain, suffering, death, lethal or harmful.
(d) Pain, suffering, distress and lasting harm.
(e) Pain, suffering, death or lasting harm.

10 *When clinical research becomes subject to A(SP)A, applications for licences are made to:*

(a) the RCVS
(b) the Home Office
(c) a university
(d) a licensed veterinary inspector
(e) a named veterinary surgeon.

16.15 MCQ answers

1. (b); 2. (d); 3. (a); 4. (e); 5. (c); 6. (e); 7. (c); 8. (e); 9. (d); 10. (b)

17

OTHER STUDY DESIGNS

Objectives

After reading this chapter readers should:

- understand the different types of studies that use secondary data analysis to answer clinical questions
- understand how to construct a decision tree and perform a treatment and testing threshold analysis
- understand the advantages and disadvantages of case series/reports and the importance of systematic data collection and accurate and detailed reporting.

This chapter will examine systematic reviews, including studies using meta-analysis. This type of study uses existing research papers to answer a clinical question. This type of study, if performed correctly, can provide the strongest evidence to support clinical judgements. Critically appraised topics have an important part to play in identifying the evidence from the published literature when a systematic review does not exist. Decision analysis using decision trees, and treatment and testing thresholds can provide useful information when there is more than one option available to the clinician and owner. Case series and case reports, although descriptive and uncontrolled, have some important functions and these are described in this section.

17.1   Systematic reviews and meta-analysis

17.1.1   *Systematic reviews*

A systematic review is a comprehensive survey of a topic in which all the primary studies of the highest level of evidence have been systematically identified, appraised and then summarized according to explicit and reproducible methodologies (Fig. 17.1). Reviews are potentially a good source of information for the busy veterinarian. The best reviews should provide unbiased summaries of all the available evidence. These are complex and difficult to produce but represent the gold standard of evidence if pro-

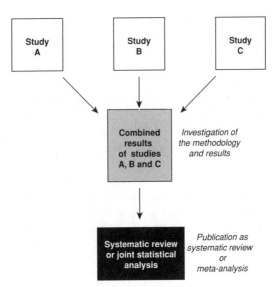

Figure 17.1 A schematic representation of the process of performing systematic reviews and meta-analyses.

duced correctly. Systematic reviews may be able to combine data from similar studies and perform a combined statistical analysis. This is called meta-analysis. Detailed protocols for systematic reviews in the form of an online handbook can be found at the Cochrane website.

The paper by Olivry and Mueller (2003) on the treatments for canine atopic dermatitis is an example of a systematic review and the abstract is given below. The method section is reproduced later to indicate the design features of a systematic review.

Evidence-based veterinary dermatology: a systematic review of the pharmacotherapy of canine atopic dermatitis (Olivry and Mueller, 2003)

Olivry T, Mueller RS, The International Task Force on Canine Atopic Dermatitis

The efficacy of pharmacological interventions used to treat canine atopic dermatitis, excluding fatty acid supplementation and allergen-specific immunotherapy, was evaluated based on the systematic review of prospective clinical trials published between 1980 and 2002. Studies were compared with regard to design characteristics (randomization generation and concealment, masking, intention-to-treat analyses and quality of enrolment of study subjects), benefit (improvement in skin lesions or pruritus scores) and harm (type, severity and frequency of adverse drug events) of the various interventions. Meta-analysis of pooled results was not possible because of heterogeneity of the drugs evaluated. Forty trials enrolling 1607 dogs were identified. There is good evidence for recommending the use of oral glucocorticoids and cyclosporin for the treatment of canine atopic dermatitis, and fair evidence for using topical triamcinolone spray, topical tacrolimus lotion, oral pentoxifylline or oral misoprostol. Insufficient evidence is available for or against recommending the prescription of oral first- and second-generation type-1 histamine receptor antagonists, tricyclic antidepressants, cyproheptadine, aspirin, Chinese herbal therapy, an homeopathic complex remedy, ascorbic acid, AHR-13268, papaverine, immune-modulating antibiotics or tranilast and topical pramoxine or capsaicin. Finally, there is fair evidence against recommending the use of oral arofylline, leukotriene synthesis inhibitors and cysteinyl leukotriene receptor antagonists.

17.1.2 Meta-analyses

A meta-analysis is a survey in which the designs of all the included studies are similar enough statistically that the results can be combined and analysed as if they were a single study. The studies should include a thorough search of the literature with defined criteria for study inclusion or exclusion.

The results of a meta-analysis are usually presented in a forest plot indicating the odds ratio and the confidence intervals of the individual and combined studies. An example of a forest plot of a meta-analysis is shown in Fig. 17.2. An odds ratio of 1 indicates no effect. An odds ratio

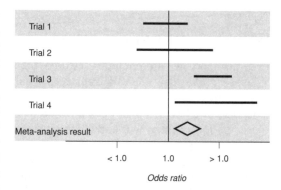

Figure 17.2 An illustration of how the results of a meta-analysis are summarized graphically.

of more than 1 indicates an improvement and an odds ratio less than 1 indicates a decline.

If all the horizontal lines indicating the 95% confidence intervals of the trial results overlap, as they do in Fig. 17.2, then the results are compatible and there is said to be homogeneity of the results. It is therefore likely that it is justifiable to combine the data from the studies as they give similar results. If they do not overlap, the results do not show heterogeneity, and this implies that the results are significantly different in some respect and should probably not be pooled. The heterogeneity may be due to differences between the trials in respect of the populations, methodology or operator bias.

Sometimes a sensitivity analysis is performed where the methods used and the studies are changed to check for consistency of the results obtained. If the results remain consistent then there is greater confidence in the reliability of the results. The abstract from a published paper using meta-analysis is reproduced below to illustrate how this technique can be used to provide evidence.

A meta-analysis review of the effects of recombinant bovine somatotropin. 1. Methodology and effects on production (Dohoo et al., 2003)

This manuscript presents the results of a review of the effects of recombinant bovine somatotropin (rBST) on milk production, milk composition, dry matter intake, and body condition score that was carried out by an expert panel established by the Canadian Veterinary Medical Association (CVMA). The panel was established by the CVMA in response to a request from Health Canada in 1998 and their report was made public in 1999. A series of meta-analyses was used to combine data on production and nutrition related parameters that were extracted from all randomized clinical trials, which had been published in peer-reviewed journals or which were provided by Health Canada, from the submission by Monsanto for registration of rBST in Canada. A companion paper will present the results of the effects of the drug on measures of health, reproductive performance, and culling parameters. Recombinant bovine somatotropin was found to increase milk production by 11.3% in primiparous cows and 15.6% in multiparous cows; although there was considerable variation from study to study. While some statistically significant effects on milk composition (% butterfat, protein, and lactose) were found, they were all very small. Treatment increased dry matter intake by an average 1.5 kg/day during the treatment period and dry matter intake remained elevated on into the first 60 days of the subsequent lactation. Despite the increase in dry matter intake, treated animals had lower body condition scores at the end of the treatment period, and the reduced scores persisted through until the start of the subsequent lactation.

17.1.3 Checklist for systematic reviews and meta-analyses

1. Will the review ask a focused question?
   In systematic reviews the question should be narrow and focused to obtain a valid outcome. Consider if the question is focused in terms of:
   > the population studied
   > the intervention given or exposure
   > the outcomes.
2. Will the review include the correct type of study?

Individual studies vary in the details of the design, choice of patients, dosages and routes of administration. These differences should be identified and related to the magnitude of the findings reported. Similar findings across a range of clinical conditions increase the strength of the finding and the effect may be more generalized than first thought. Consider if the included studies addressed the question: Had they used an appropriate study design?

3. Will you identify all the relevant studies?
   Research papers are the raw data of a review and need to be selected with care. The concern is that the review may contain a biased sample of papers. The details of the search should be described: which databases were searched and what key terms were used in the search.

4. Will publication bias be taken into account?
   Papers that report positive findings have a higher chance of publication than those which conclude that a new treatment is ineffective. This may bias the conclusion.

5. What explicit guidelines and inclusion and exclusion criteria will be used to determine which findings to include in the review stated?
   Will selection bias be minimized (e.g. by not only selecting studies with positive findings)?

6. Will you assess the quality of the included studies?
   Not all research studies are well designed and conducted. Selection is therefore important. Assessment of the quality and the strength of each paper is important. Are the criteria for assessment explicit and sensible? How will you handle missing information?

7. Can the results of the studies be combined in a meta-analysis?
   Some variation in the results can be accounted for by chance. However, heterogeneity of effect can occur due to differences in design. Studies which share design features should have broadly similar results.

Whenever there is evidence of heterogeneity the process summarizing the studies with a singe measure becomes doubtful. Were the results of each study similar (was there homogeneity or heterogeneity)? Were the study designs similar?

8. How will the results be presented?

The results of individual studies can be presented in a table or figure to allow the reader to judge whether on balance they give a consistent answer. In a meta-analysis the results, if combined, must use appropriate and explicit statistical techniques:

- Will *P* values be given?
- Will confidence intervals be given?

Poorer quality studies may be accommodated by using a weighting system: the worse the study, the lower the weighting. Alternatively a sensitivity analysis is sometimes performed where the quality of the study to be included is increased and the effect on the result observed. If broadly the same result is obtained across a range of quality thresholds then the findings can be accepted.

17.1.4　Methods section of a systematic review

Below is the methods section of the paper by Olivry and Mueller on canine atopic dermatitis, which provides an excellent example of how the principles of ranking studies can be applied.

Methods (Olivry and Mueller, 2003)

Search strategy

In order to retrieve all clinical trials enrolling canine patients with atopic dermatitis (AD), a wide electronic search was carried out using the MEDLINE database. A broad query was done with the following user string: (dog OR dogs OR canine) and (atop* OR pruritus) with a limit set from 1980 to 2002. A second focused search was made with the same string limited to the 'therapy' category of the clinical queries using research methodology filters. To increase the

retrieval of additional veterinary medical citations, both CAB ABSTRACT and ISI Web of Science databases were queried using the following string: (atopy or atopic or pruritus) and (dog or dogs or canine). The search was limited to articles published after 1980. The four volumes of *Advances in Veterinary Dermatology*, which include peer-reviewed original articles presented at previous World Congresses of Veterinary Dermatology, were hand-searched for studies pertinent to this review. Similarly, the bibliographies of all articles and book chapters covering treatment of canine AD or pruritus were scanned for additional relevant citations. Finally, a message was posted on the Vetderm listserv (1 November 2002) to request identification and sharing of clinical trials recently accepted for publication in peer-reviewed journals.

Selection of studies

This systematic analysis was restricted to prospective clinical trials published in peer-reviewed veterinary or medical journals from 1980 to 2002. There was no limitation based on language of publication. Clinical trials were included only if study participants included at least five dogs with AD, this disease being defined as 'a genetically predisposed inflammatory and pruritic allergic skin disease with characteristic clinical features and associated most commonly with IgE antibodies to environmental allergens'.

Only clinical trials that evaluated pharmacological interventions aimed at the treatment of AD were included in this systematic review. Also, studies needed to report at least one clinical outcome to exclude those that solely described biological changes after pharmacological intervention.

Data extraction

Clinical trials that satisfied inclusion criteria were reviewed independently by the leading authors (TO and RSM) who assessed quality of study design, participants' characteristics, details of interventions and outcome measures. Data were abstracted in tabular form. Results of the review were compared, and where differences were noted, they were discussed and reconciled.

Quality assessment

Assessment of methodological quality

Three parameters were addressed to determine the risk for biased estimates of treatment effect in the included studies:

1. randomization, method of generation and concealment of allocation to treatment groups;
2. masking, blinding of observers (e.g. clinicians) and participants (e.g. owners) to the treatment allocation;
3. loss-to-follow-up, presence of dropouts and withdrawals and intention-to-treat (ITT) analyses. The latter term denotes the performance of statistical analyses on all subjects entered in the trial, whether or not they had actually received the intervention and completed the study. ITT analyses are believed to prevent overestimation of treatment efficacy in case of substantial withdrawal of study subjects due to adverse drug events.

These three components were graded in accordance to the recommendations of the Cochrane Skin Group as 'adequate', 'unclear' or 'inadequate'. When trials were not randomized, 'none' was the qualifier provided for the randomization parameter. When statistical analyses were not performed, a specific mention of this was written.

An overall grade of evidence quality, based on the parameters discussed above and the number of subjects entered in active treatment groups, was provided for each study as follows:

(A) blinded randomized controlled trial (control with either active drug or placebo);
(B) controlled trial lacking either blinding or randomization;
(C) open, uncontrolled trial;
(D) cohort study, case-control analytic study, descriptive study, case report:

(1) > 50 subjects per group,
(2) 20–50 subjects per group,
(3) 10–19 subjects per group,
(4) < 10 subjects per group.

Example: the quality of evidence of a blinded RCT enrolling 30 subjects (15 in each group), will be graded A3, that of an open trial of 25 dogs will be C2.

Of note is that such grading scheme could be misleading on rare occasions. Indeed, one could assume that a large blinded RCT (AI) with poorly defined outcome measures would provide evidence of higher quality than that of a well-designed yet smaller nonblinded RCT (B2). Readers are urged to use caution whenever making such assumptions.

Assessment of subject enrolment quality

For each of the eligible studies, criteria for inclusion of subjects were reviewed to assess the method of diagnosis of AD in comparison with currently accepted standards. The quality of subject selection was evaluated for each trial as follows:

- well-characterized was the term used when only patients with AD were entered in the study, and sufficient details on the methods of diagnosis of AD (clinical signs, rule-out of concurrent or resembling skin diseases, etc.) were provided to allow comparison with current standards
- poorly-characterized was used when participant selection criteria were vague (e.g. uncharacterized 'allergic pruritus'), and insufficient details of the diagnostic work-up were provided
- fairly-characterized was used for intermediate situations.

Assessment of outcome measures

Whenever possible, the following four outcome measures were calculated from reported study data to compare efficacy between interventions: (i) percentage of reduction from baseline of skin lesion scores; (ii) percentage of reduction from baseline of pruritus scores; (iii) percentage of dogs achieving 50% or greater reduction from baseline of skin lesion scores; (iv) percentage of dogs achieving 50% or greater reduction from baseline of pruritus scores.

A 50% reduction from baseline of pruritus or lesion scores is believed to represent a clinically relevant threshold above which both clinicians and owners are satisfied with treatment effect. This benchmark also mirrors the 'good-to-excellent efficacy' subjective outcome measure that was employed in most clinical trials reported in the early 1990s.

When published information was insufficient to permit abstraction of the four outcome measures described above, authors of recently published RCTs were contacted with a request to supply individual scores of all study subjects. Missing data were replaced in accordance to the 'last-value-carry forward' rule. For non-RCT studies published more than five years ago for which such specific measures were not provided, author-reported variables were quoted. Finally, all published adverse effects were collated and assessed for evaluation of treatment harm.

Meta-analysis of randomized controlled trials

Because there were few trials investigating the same intervention, results were not presented fully in many articles, enrolment of study subjects was heterogeneous, and only few RCTs overall were available, meta-analysis of pooled results was not considered appropriate.

Reporting of qualitative results

Pharmacological interventions were grouped in different sections based on similar mechanisms of drug action. Study design, patient enrolment quality, nature of interventions and main out-come measures were summarized in narrative and/or tabular forms.

A recommendation of use of these drugs for treatment of canine AD will be proposed following careful scrutiny of the evidence of efficacy and harm of the interventions reported in the various sections. The strength of recommendation qualifier was modified from the 1996 report of the US Preventive Services Task Force as either good or fair evidence for use of the medication, insufficient evidence for/against use of the medication or fair or good evidence against use of the medication. The basis for such recommendation statements will be as follows:

1. When more than one study, including at least one blinded RCT, supports the high efficacy of the drug tested, there is 'good' evidence 'for' recommending the use of this medication.
2. When at least one blinded RCT provides support of medium to high efficacy of the drug investigated, there will be 'fair' evidence 'for' recommending the use of that drug.
3. When blinded RCTs are not available, or when multiple studies yield controversial evidence of treatment effect, it will be concluded that there is 'insufficient' evidence 'for/against' recommending prescription of the medication tested.
4. When at least one blinded RCT provides evidence of lack of efficacy, or efficacy associated with common harmful events, there is 'fair' evidence 'against' recommending the use of this medication.
5. When more than one study, including at least one blinded RCT, supports the lack of efficacy of the drug tested, or supports any efficacy but with unacceptable side effects, there is 'good' evidence 'against' recommending the use of drug evaluated.

17.2   Critically appraised topics

A critically appraised topic (CAT) is a short summary of the evidence for a focused clinical question when a systematic review does not exist. CATs are normally published on dedicated websites. The preparation of a CAT enables this information to be shared between clinicians and is subject to varying degrees of peer review. Standard protocols have been produced regarding the format of CATS. Some evidence-based medicine centres use the acronym POEM (Patient Orientated Evidence that Matters) as an alternative to CAT. An example of the process is given by the CAT on ovariectomy in the bitch and the occurrence of mammary tumours below.

17.2.1   *Ovariectomy of bitches reduces the incidence of mammary tumours*

Three part question

In: healthy bitches – breed or age unspecified (population)
Does: ovariectomy (intervention)
Reduce: the incidence of mammary carcinomas (outcome)?

Clinical scenario

A client presents a bitch for vaccination and asks for advice on whether ovariectomy will reduce the incidence of mammary tumours.

Author:
Dr Mark Holmes 8/9/2005 (not refereed)
University of Cambridge, Department of Veterinary Medicine

Search strategy:
Pubmed/Medline 1966–Aug 2005)
(canine and mammary and cancer and incidence)

Search outcome:
A total of 181 papers retrieved. Sixteen papers described studies which provided information relevant to the question (Arnesen et al., 1995; Bastianello, 1983; Dobson et al., 2002;

Egenvall et al., 2005; Else and Hannant, 1979; MacVean et al., 1978; Moe, 2001; Mulligan, 1975; O'Brien et al., 2000; Perez Alenza et al., 2000; Richards et al., 2001; Rostami et al., 1994; Schneider, 1970; Schneider et al., 1969; Sonnenschein et al., 1991; Sorenmo, 2003). Three papers provided specific data resulting from studies using appropriate methodology.

Relevant papers:
Schneider, R., Dorn, C.R., Taylor, D.O., 1969, Factors influencing canine mammary cancer development and postsurgical survival. J Natl Cancer Inst 43, 1249–1261.

Sonnenschein, E.G., Glickman, L.T., Goldschmidt, M.H., McKee, L.J., 1991, Body conformation, diet, and risk of breast cancer in pet dogs: a case-control study. Am J Epidemiol 133, 694–703

Richards, H.G., McNeil, P.E., Thompson, H., Reid, S.W., 2001, An epidemiological analysis of a canine-biopsies database compiled by a diagnostic histopathology service. Prev Vet Med 51, 125–136.

Conclusion

Clients should be advised that there is strong evidence that ovariectomy reduces the risk of bitches developing malignant mammary neoplasia later in life. The odds of developing cancer are highly likely to be one third (or better) than those of entire bitches. In the UK we estimate the lifetime probability of mammary neoplasia in entire bitches to be about 8% (or 1 in 13). A conservative estimate for the effect of spaying (at any age) is that we avoid one death resulting from mammary malignancy for every 20 bitches spayed.

Furthermore there is good evidence that spaying before the age of 1 yr considerably reduces the risk (one paper indicates that early neutering reduces the risk to 1/100 that of entire bitches).

Author, Date, Country	Study type	Population[1]	Case definition	Controls	Numbers	Key results[2]	Clinical interpretation[3]
Scneider et al. 1969 USA	Case-control	Diagnostic submissions from veterinary practice	Histopathological	Non-cancer diagnoses of histopathological submissions. Matched on breed and age	Neutered cases: 24 Entire cases: 63 Neutered controls: 64 Entire controls: 23	Odds Ratio: 0.14 (95% CI 0.07–0.27)[4]	Estimated ARR based on 8% lifetime risk[5]: 6.8% (CI 5.7–7.4%) Estimated NNT 15 (CI 14–18)
Sonnenschein et al. 1991 USA	Case-control	Diagnostic submissions from veterinary practice	Histopathological	Two groups, one with non-mammary tumours, the other based on non-neoplastic diagnoses. Matched on age and breed.	*Non-cancer controls* Neutered cases: 56 Entire cases: 94 Neutered controls: 107 Entire controls: 40 *Cancer controls* Neutered cases: 56 Entire cases: 94 Neutered controls: 107 Entire controls: 40	Odds Ratio: 0.39 (95% CI 0.24–0.63)[6] Odds Ratio: 0.22 (95% CI 0.14–0.36)	Estimated ARR based on 8% lifetime risk: 6.1% (CI 5.0–6.8%) Estimated NNT 16 (CI 15–20) Estimated ARR based on 8% lifetime risk: 4.7% (CI 2.8–6.0%) Estimated NNT 21 (CI 17–36)
Richards et al. 2001 UK	Case-control	Diagnostic submissions from veterinary practice	Histopathological	Non-cancer diagnoses of histopathological submissions. Matched on breed and age	Break down of mammary tumour numbers not provided. 2018 cases of mammary neoplasia. Numbers for all female diagnoses and controls: Neutered: 4920 Entire: 7005	Found no significant difference in the odds ratio for a diagnosis of neoplasia in mammary gland samples from intact or neutered females.	Ovariectomy does not affect the incidence of mammary neoplasia in the dog.[7]

Notes:

[1]The populations for all the cases and controls used in these studies comprised of animals presented to general veterinary practices, specialist veterinary practices or university veterinary hospitals. As such they may may not represent the entire canine population due to 'referral' bias. However they might reasonably be expected to represent the population for which the risk is being assessed (i.e. those animals owned by clients presenting their pets at a veterinary practice for consideration for neutering).

[2]These results are all independently derived from raw data extracted from the papers. This process ignores or discards any statistical stratification methodology that may have been used by the authors (e.g. techniques that account for bias resulting from uneven distribution of factors that may also influence tumour incidence such as age or breed). They do however enable simple comparison of the overall effects of ovariectomy between the papers. These figures will not be any more accurate than those published. They will not be any more accurate than those published.

[3] It should be noted that risk reduction is not conventionally derived from odds ratios (OR) provided from case control studies. These figures are provided as an aid to their use in the clinical decision making process and cannot be relied upon to provide definitive evidence of the true risks in the general population. In these papers the OR represents the odds that a case of malignant mammary neoplasia has been spayed. If there are no other factors that might be anticipated to influence this association it may be considered reasonable to invert the retrospective observation into a prospective risk ratio for the spayed or entire groups.

The NNT (number needed to treat) is a figure representing the number of animals that would need to receive the intervention (ovariectomy in this case) in order to have one animal with a favourable outcome (i.e. to prevent one animal developing a malignant mammary tumour).

[4] This paper reported results in the form of relative risks. A Mantel-Haenszel analysis was performed in order to test the significance of the relative risks (this is a method which takes account of factors which influence the likelihood of the outcome including the sparing effect of test variables and is an alternative approach to using logistic regression). The absence of the presentation of much of the raw data makes interpretation of this paper difficult. This is the most widely quoted paper on the mammary malignancy sparing effect of ovariectomy. The key result reported in this paper is a relative risk of 0.12 for all neutered cases. The paper also attempts to estimate the relative risks of ovariectomy prior to the first season (1 case, 26 controls: relative risk reported as 0.05), before the second season (3 cases, 11 controls: relative risk reported as 0.08), and in bitches after two or more seasons (20 cases, 25 controls: relative risk reported as 0.26). Although this represents some evidence of the sparing effect of early neutering the numbers are insufficient for accurate quantification of risk reduction although these figures are frequently used in the secondary literature.

[5] A comprehensive study performed in Sweden on over 80,000 insured female dogs reported a case fatality rate resulting from mammary neoplasia for a cohort of births between 1992 and 1993 of 8% (Egenvall et al., 2005). Routine neutering is rarely performed in Sweden. Some of the bitches in the study population will have been spayed for medical reasons (e.g. pyometra) although it is reasonable to assume this will have been performed after two or more oestruses.

An estimated lifetime risk of 2% was obtained from a paper describing canine neoplasia rates in the UK which reported a rate of 178 mammary tumours (malignant or unspecified) per 100,000 per year assuming an average lifespan of 11 years (Dobson et al., 2002). This paper did attempt to normalise the results to represent the overall UK dog population. It is important to note that a considerable proportion of these animals are likely to have been neutered at an early age which will have influenced the incidence.

A study carried out in Norway (Moe, 2001) where routine neutering is not commonplace reported population-based incidence rates of 35, 3.9, and 18 cases of malignant mammary tumours per 1000 female dogs per year in boxers, Bernese mountain dogs and bichon frise respectively. The author estimates that the lifetime risk may be as high as 40% in entire boxer bitches. This figure would lead to an absolute risk reduction of approximately 34% with an NNT of 3.

[6] This paper provides the strongest evidence of the effect of age or number of oestruses before ovariectomy. The paper reports odds ratios (OR) for ovariectomy up to 1 yr of 0.01 (for boths sets of controls); for ovariectomy at 1.1–2.5 yrs the ORs were 0.11 and 0.13 for the cancer controls and non-cancer controls respectively; and for ovariectomy at 2.6–5 yrs the OR was 0.3 for the cancer controls. Independent derivation of these figures was not possible from the data provided.

[7] This is a surprising negative finding in what appears to be a well-conducted study comparable to the others. It is conceivable, although perhaps unlikely, that there were a large number of cases in bitches neutered at ages greater than 2.5 yrs. Unfortunately the authors did not have access to the age at which the cases were neutered.

17.3 Decision analysis

Optimal decision making requires veterinary surgeons to identify all possible strategies, accurately predict the probability of future events, and balance the risks and benefits of each possible action in consultation with the client. Decision analysis is a formalization of the decision-making process. The decision tree is a flow diagram that outlines the outcomes that could follow each potential decision and calculates the probability and value of each event.

17.3.1 Decision trees

Decision analysis provides a methodology to quantify the outcomes of decisions so that the best-informed choice, based on the best external evidence and the owners' preferred values, can be identified. An appropriate and valid decision tree is the best technique for evidence-based decision making. It recognizes the owners' value system, can be quantitatively analysed and makes the clinical reasoning behind a decision explicit.

A decision tree consists of nodes, which describe decisions, chances and outcomes. The tree is used to illustrate the strategies available to the veterinary surgeon and the likelihood of each outcome if a particular decision is made. Objective estimates of the outcomes may be derived from published research studies, records or subjective estimates.

Decision trees are composed of decision nodes, chance nodes, terminal nodes and utilities.

Decision nodes

Decision nodes indicate a conscious decision between two or more options. They are often depicted as squares in diagrams of decision trees.

Chance nodes

No decisions are made at a chance node but likelihoods are attached to each outcome derived from a chance node. The likelihoods or probabilities of the outcomes emanating from a chance node add up to 1.0 or 100%, respectively.

Chance nodes are often depicted as circles in diagrams of decision trees.

Terminal nodes

Terminal nodes are often represented as triangles or squares where no more decisions are taken. Utilities are attached to these terminal nodes to indicate the value attached to the outcome by the owner.

Utilities

Utilities use a 0–1 scale that reflects how important the outcome is to the owner. They are subjective in character. The best utility is given a value of 1.0 and the worst utility a value of 0.0. Every other outcome receives an intermediate score reflecting its relative value to the owner when compared to the two extremes. Utility scores do not have to add up to a specific number. The values should be rational and consistent. The utility then has to be multiplied by the probability of the outcome for which it has been defined to produce the expected utility. The expected utility with the highest value is the best option. Deciding on utilities in veterinary medicine can be difficult as the animal's welfare must be safeguarded at all costs. However, it is important that the owner is able to express a preference. The choice of a utility is likely to be a consensus between veterinary surgeon and owner.

17.3.2 Solving the decision tree

In order to identify the outcome with the highest expected utility, the probability of the terminal outcome has to be computed. This is accomplished by identifying each probability on the pathway from the terminal node to the root of the tree. These probabilities multiplied together give the probability of the outcome. If all the probabilities of the terminal nodes are added together they should come to 1.0 if likelihoods have been used, or 100% if probabilities have been used. This is a useful check on mathematical accuracy. The probability of the outcome is then multiplied by the utility to compute the expected utility. Outcomes in many cases are still a matter of chance and it is important that the owner understands that the outcome with the highest expected utility may not be achieved.

17.3.3 Sensitivity analysis

Sensitivity analysis is performed to establish the relative importance of particular variables. If a variable is changed, how much does it have to be changed to make a significant difference to the outcome? In one-way sensitivity analysis the value of one variable is changed. In two- and three-way sensitivity analysis two or three variable values, respectively, are changed simultaneously. When we use estimated values (e.g. an estimated prevalence) sensitivity analysis is a good way of working out how accurate the estimates need to be.

17.3.4 Constructing a decision tree

The construction of a decision tree and the decision analysis proceeds by the following steps:

1. The tree is composed of clinical decisions for which all the relevant outcomes are defined.
2. A probability is attached to each of the outcomes for the decision.
3. The probability of the terminal outcome is the product of the probabilities of the preceding outcomes.
4. A utility is attached to the terminal outcome.
5. The option with the highest expected utility is selected.
6. The effect of changing any estimated probabilities and utilities can be assessed by changing their values and observing the effect on outcome values (sensitivity analysis).

Once the tree has been constructed check that:

- all the important treatment options and outcomes of these options (good and bad) are included in the construction of the tree.
- the probabilities attached to the outcomes are based on the best evidence and are credible.
- the utilities are credible.
- if estimates were used, were outcome utilities generated for a credible range of values?

Decision trees are effectively mathematical models that enable us to look at the final outcome arising from a particular decision (or set of decisions). The construction of a decision tree requires detailed information on the probabilities of the various outcomes and the utility of the outcome to the patient. A utility is a value that is placed on the outcome by the owner. That value may not be simply economic but may include the quality of life for the animal. The expected utility for each branch of the decision tree can be calculated from the probability of the outcome and the utility of the outcome. By examining the utilities of each terminal branch of the decision tree the best option can be identified to optimize the patient's welfare and/or the owner's wishes.

17.3.5 Obtaining utility values from clients and owners

Utilities represent an owner's quantitative measure for a particular outcome. The utilities that are assigned to each of the outcomes are very subjective. They are not entities that we think of in numerical terms and so various techniques have been developed to aid their generation.

Visual analogue scales

Visual analogue scales are used to assist the owner. It is found that humans tend to avoid placing a mark at the extremes of the scales and thereby introduce a bias.

Time trade-off

The owner is presented with a trade-off between the quality of life of the patient and the length of life left in time of the patient.

Consider two health states: perfectly healthy and impaired health status.

Assume:

time (healthy) × utility (healthy) = time (impaired) × utility (impaired)

Time trade establishes that 4 years lived with a utility of 0.5 is equivalent to 2 years with a perfect utility of 1.0. By getting the owner to choose relative time equivalences we are able to obtain the utility value. For example, if a dog is faced with a potential lifetime of 4 years with a severe limp, what reduction of lifetime would you (the owner) be willing to accept for the dog to have perfect health?

Let us assume that the owner says a reduction of 1 year (i.e. 3 years without a limp is equivalent to 4 years with a limp):

4 − 1(healthy time) × 1(healthy utility) = 4(impaired time) × (impaired utility)

$$(\text{impaired utility}) = \frac{(4-1)}{4} = \frac{3}{4} = 0.75$$

The utility value calculated from the owner's view on the severe limp is 0.75.

Standard gamble

In this scenario the owner is forced to choose between accepting a certain health state for the animal or taking a gamble on a better outcome while risking the worst outcome. The owner is presented with two doors. Behind door 1 is the certain outcome for an intermediate health state for which the utility is required from the patient. Behind door 2 are two hypothetical outcomes: the best possible outcome (complete recovery) and the worst possible outcome (death). The owner has to select which door to choose. By changing the probabilities of the two outcomes behind door 2 it is possible to reach a point where the owner finds it difficult to make a choice between door 1 and door 2. At this point the utility is equal to the probability of the best outcome behind door 2. For example, most of us would open the second door if the likelihood of complete cure was 99.9% and most of us would not open the second door if there were a 90% chance of death.

17.3.6   Decision analysis tree for therapeutic decisions

Figure 17.3 illustrates a decision tree for a condition that has both a surgical and a medical option. In this example successful surgery with no pain or deformity is the best utility (1.0) and an outcome with pain and deformity is the worst utility (0.0). Multiplying the probability of each outcome with the utility of each outcome produces the expected utility for each outcome. Adding all the expected utilities of the medical outcomes together gives the expected utility of the medical option, in this instance 0.525. Adding all the expected utilities of the surgical outcomes together gives the expected utility of the surgical option, in this instance 0.830. The conclusion is that the outcome of the surgical option is likely to be better (Cockcroft and Holmes, 2003).

Figure 17.4 is a decision tree that was constructed to estimate the lifespan that might be expected for a dog presented with cryptorchidism at 1 year of age if it underwent a preventive orchidectomy or if it did not (Peters and van Sluis, 2002). The expected utility value is expressed in terms of expected survival time in years. The decision tree indicates there is no significant difference in the expected lifespan. The risk of anaesthetic or surgical complications is similar to the risk of morbidity and mortality due to testicular tumour. A decision tree is only a tool to help the clinician to estimate the risks of treatment, and other important factors to consider before making a decision are the behavioural changes induced

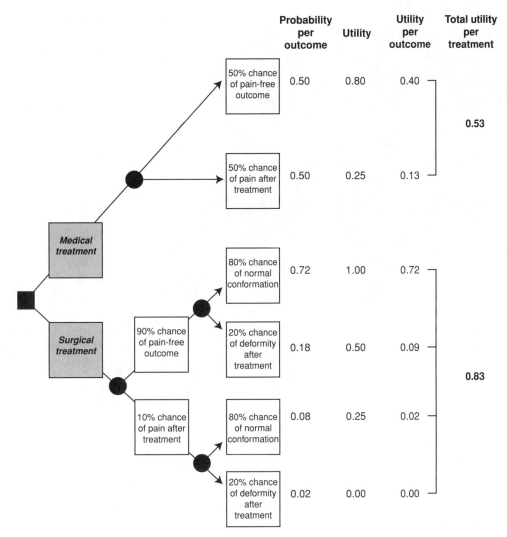

	Probability per outcome	Utility	Utility per outcome	Total utility per treatment
50% chance of pain-free outcome	0.50	0.80	0.40	
50% chance of pain after treatment	0.50	0.25	0.13	0.53
80% chance of normal conformation	0.72	1.00	0.72	
20% chance of deformity after treatment	0.18	0.50	0.09	
80% chance of normal conformation	0.08	0.25	0.02	0.83
20% chance of deformity after treatment	0.02	0.00	0.00	

Figure 17.3 A decision tree illustrating the analysis of a hypothetical decision to choose between a medical and a surgical treatment.

by castration and the increased risk of obesity. Dog owners should be informed about these side effects. Another consideration is that cryptorchidism is considered to be inherited and that castration may therefore be advisable to prevent breeding from affected animals. Because the decision tree indicates that orchidectomy would not make a significant difference to the life expectancy, it would seem advisable to monitor a

cryptorchid dog frequently for the development of a testicular tumour and operate only when one is suspected.

17.3.7 Decision analysis tree for economic decisions

Canine gastric dilatation (GDV) is an acute condition affecting primarily large and giant breeds of

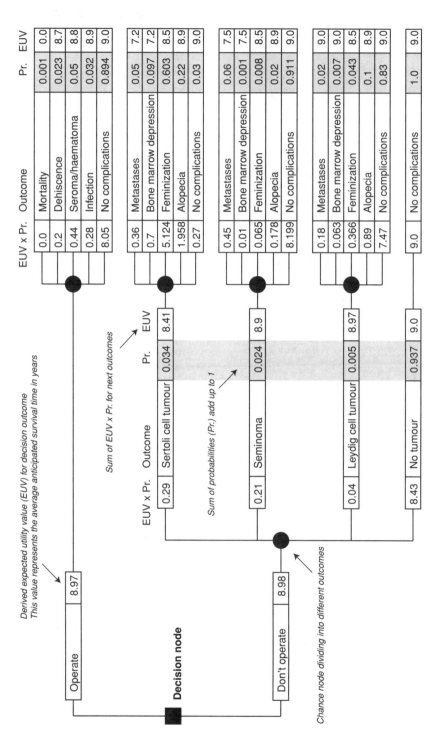

Figure 17.4 Decision tree for preventive orchidectomy in a cryptorchid dog. The tree has two branches: 'operate' and 'don't operate'. The branch 'don't operate' has four possibilities: 'Sertoli cell tumour', 'seminoma', 'Leydig cell tumour' and 'no tumour'. The calculation of the expected utility values (EUV) (expected survival time in years when the decision is made) of each branch starts on the right and proceeds to the left. The EUV of the possibilities 'operate', 'Sertoli cell tumour', 'seminoma' and 'Leydig cell tumour' are calculated by summing the products of the EUV and the probability of each possible outcome. For the branch 'operate', this yields the EUV of this branch. The EUV of the branch 'don't operate' is calculated by summing the products of the EUV and the probability of each possibility. The probabilities of 'Sertoli cell tumour', 'seminoma' and 'Leydig cell tumour' are derived from the literature. The probability of the remaining possibility 'no tumour' is 1 minus the sum of the other probabilities in the same branch. Pr., probability; ■, decision; ●, chance. From Peters and van Sluis (2002).

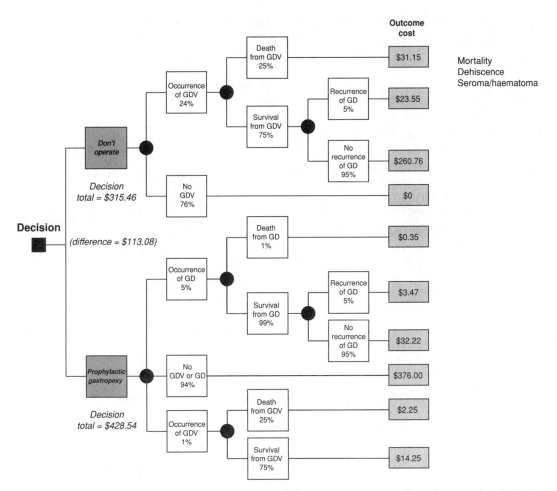

Figure 17.5 Example of a decision tree for prophylactic gastropexy solved for cost for the Irish Setter (lifetime probability of GDV = 0.249). Assumptions were cost of prophylactic gastropexy US$ 400, cost of treatment for GDV US$ 1500 if a dog survived, cost of treatment US$ 500 if a dog died and cost of treatment for gastric dilatation without volvulus US$ 300.■, decision; ●, chance. From Ward et al. (2003).

dog. It is characterized by accumulations of gas in the stomach and varying degrees of gastric malposition, leading to increased intragastric pressure, cardiogenic shock and (often) death. Ward et al. (2003) used a decision tree to determine the cost benefit of performing prophylactic gastropexy in the Irish Setter to avoid the condition (Fig. 17.5). The expected excess expense associated with prophylactic gastropexy was US$-113.08, suggesting that the best course of action using cost alone as the outcome measure was not to perform a prophylactic gastropexy using the current cost of the procedure. In addition to the cost outcome decision tree, a decision tree indicating the impact of gastropexy on the reduction in the lifetime probability of death from GDV (6.3 to 0.3%, a 20-fold reduction in the Red Setter) allows veterinarians and owners to make informed choices. Additional ethical issues in show animals may be additional factors to consider.

17.3.8   *Testing and treating thresholds*

Decision analysis can be used to decide if a patient should undergo a diagnostic test and/or treatment. In this analysis, the probability of disease in a patient (the pre-test probability, derived from the prevalence) is compared to the testing threshold value and the treatment threshold value. Values for the following five factors are required to compute the testing and treatment thresholds:

- benefit of therapy
- risk or cost of therapy
- risk of the test
- sensitivity of the test
- specificity of the test

The values of the benefit, risk of therapy and risk of test can be in terms of either cost (£) or the likelihood of a favourable outcome (0–1.0):

The values for the testing and treating thresholds are then compared to the patient pre-test likelihood (range 0–1.0).

There are three possible outcomes:

1. Probability of disease in the patient is below the testing threshold.
   With this result both the treatment and the test should be withheld. The risk or cost of the test outweighs the benefit of the test diagnostic information.
2. Probability of disease in the patient is between the testing and treating threshold (the testing band)
   The test should be performed and treatment guided by the test result.
3. Probability of disease in the patient is above the treating threshold
   Treatment should be given without testing, as the diagnostic test result will not change the action.

These outcomes are illustrated in Fig. 17.6.

Worked veterinary examples are provided by Smith (1991). Treatment and testing thresholds

$$\text{testing threshold} = \frac{((1 - \text{specificity}) \times \text{risk of therapy}) + \text{risk of test}}{((1 - \text{specificity}) \times \text{risk of therapy}) + (\text{sensitivity} \times \text{benefit of therapy})}$$

$$\text{treatment threshold} = \frac{(\text{specificity} \times \text{risk of therapy}) - \text{risk of test}}{(\text{specificity} \times \text{risk of therapy}) + ((1 - \text{sensitivity}) \times \text{benefit of therapy})}$$

The values obtained whether using costs or likelihoods are in the range 0–1.0.

are covered in considerable detail by Friedland and Bent (1998).

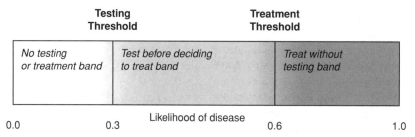

Figure 17.6 A diagrammatic representation of thresholds, and testing and treatment bands.

17.4 Case series and case reports

A large proportion of the veterinary literature consists of case reports or case series. A case report is a report on a single patient. A case series is a collection of case reports on the treatment of a condition or a clinical description of a condition.

A case report describes the presentation and/or course of a disease. It may be a novel presentation or an undocumented course of a familiar disease or a description of a rare disease. The purpose of the report is to present a particular history, clinical description, diagnosis, treatment or prognosis to the veterinary profession.

A case series can provide descriptive quantitative data that are useful in identifying the range and the frequencies of presentations that may be encountered. Descriptions of treatments and associated potential risk factors should be viewed with extreme caution and used to generate hypotheses only.

Case series and case reports have no statistical validity since there is no control group but they may be helpful if other sources of evidence are not available with regard to a rare condition. Case reports and case series are not usually thought of as research, and are traditionally regarded as the lowest form of evidence. However, in the absence of other sources of information they have an important part to play in the acquisition of evidence.

Case reports are not a valid contribution to the literature unless they (Mason 1995):

- report the unique or nearly unique case which represents a previously undescribed disease in a particular species or defined geographical area or
- report an unreported association of two or more diseases or a disease and risk factor or report an unusual variant of a well-recognized disease.

17.4.1 Advantages

- Rare complications of interventions may be reported that may not be documented in other research trials.
- New and emerging diseases may be first described as a case report, e.g. BSE.
- They may serve as early indicators of novel developments, risks, and diagnostic and therapeutic options.
- They are hypothesis generating not hypothesis proving.

17.4.2 Disadvantages

- The intervention described may not have influenced the outcome.
- There may be harm attached to the intervention.
- The description may be atypical of the rare disease.
- There may be a publication bias in that promising or interesting interventions are published, whereas less interesting or unpromising ones are not.
- The conclusions from these reports should be interpreted with maximum caution.

Case reports can be prospective or retrospective. It is important that a systematic approach to data collection is applied and that sufficient detail is provided to characterize the individuals and populations accurately. Careful consideration should be given to whether a case report or case series is the best approach. Limited research time may be more appropriately spent using more powerful research designs.

17.5 References

Arnesen K, Gamlem H, Glattre E, Moe L, Nordstoga K (1995) [Registration of canine cancer]. *Tidsskr Nor Laegeforen* 115, 714–717.

Bastianello SS (1983) A survey on neoplasia in domestic species over a 40-year period from 1935 to 1974 in the Republic of South Africa. VI. Tumours occurring in dogs. *Onderstepoort J Vet Res* 50, 199–220.

Cockcroft PD, Holmes M (2003) Decision analysis, models and economics as evidence. In: *Handbook of*

Evidence-based Veterinary Medicine, Blackwell Publishing, Oxford, p 162.

Dobson JM, Samuel S, Milstein H, Rogers K, Wood JL (2002) Canine neoplasia in the UK: estimates of incidence rates from a population of insured dogs. *J Small Anim Pract* **43**, 240–246.

Dohoo IR, Leslie K, DesCoteaux L, Fredeen A, Dowling P, Preston A, Shewfelt W (2003) A meta-analysis review of the effects of recombinant bovine somatotropin. 1. Methodology and effects on production. *Can. J. Vet. Res.* **67**(4): 241–51.

Egenvall A, Bonnett BN, Ohagen P, Olson P, Hedhammar A, von Euler H (2005) Incidence of and survival after mammary tumors in a population of over 80,000 insured female dogs in Sweden from 1995 to 2002. *Prev Vet Med* **69**, 109–127.

Else RW, Hannant D (1979) Some epidemiological aspects of mammary neoplasia in the bitch. *Vet Rec* **104**, 296–304.

Friedland DJ, Bent AR (1998) Treatment and testing thresholds. In: *Evidence-Based Medicine: A Framework for Clinical Practice*, Friedland DJ (ed.), Lange Medical Books/McGraw-Hill, New York, pp 59–60.

MacVean DW, Monlux AW, Anderson PS, Jr, Silberg SL, Roszel JF (1978) Frequency of canine and feline tumors in a defined population. *Vet Pathol* **15**, 700–715.

Mason I (1995) Writing and publishing a paper in a veterinary journal. *J. Small Anim. Pract.* **36**(5): 214–20.

Moe L (2001) Population-based incidence of mammary tumours in some dog breeds. *J Reprod Fertil Suppl* **57**, 439–43.

Mulligan RM (1975) Mammary cancer in the dog: a study of 120 cases. *Am J Vet Res* **36**, 1391–1396.

O'Brien DJ, Kaneene JB, Getis A, Lloyd JW, Swanson GM, Leader RW (2000) Spatial and temporal comparison of selected cancers in dogs and humans, Michigan, USA, 1964–1994. *Prev Vet Med* **47**, 187–204.

Olivry T, Mueller RS (2003) Evidence-based dermatology: a systematic review of the pharmacotherapy of canine atopic dermatitis. *Vet. Dermatol.* **14**: 121–46.

Perez Alenza MD, Pena L, del Castillo N, Nieto, AI (2000) Factors influencing the incidence and prognosis of canine mammary tumours. *J Small Anim Pract* **41**, 287–291.

Peters MAJ, van Sluis FJ (2002) Decision analysis tree for deciding whether to remove an undescended testis from a young dog. *Vet. Rec.* **150**(13): 408–11.

Richards HG, McNeil PE, Thompson H, Reid SW (2001) An epidemiological analysis of a canine-biopsies database compiled by a diagnostic histopathology service. *Prev Vet Med* **51**, 125–136.

Rostami M, Tateyama S, Uchida K, Naitou H, Yamaguchi R, Otsuka H (1994) Tumors in domestic animals examined during a ten-year period (1980 to 1989) at Miyazaki University. *J Vet Med Sci* **56**, 403–405.

Schneider R (1970) Comparison of age, sex, and incidence rates in human and canine breast cancer. *Cancer* **26**, 419–426.

Schneider R, Dorn CR, Taylor DO (1969) Factors influencing canine mammary cancer development and postsurgical survival. *J Natl Cancer Inst* **43**, 1249–1261.

Sonnenschein EG, Glickman LT, Goldschmidt MH, McKee LJ (1991) Body conformation, diet, and risk of breast cancer in pet dogs: a case-control study. *Am J Epidemiol* **133**, 694–703.

Sorenmo K (2003) Canine mammary gland tumors. *Vet Clin North Am Small Anim Pract* **33**, 573–596.

Ward MP, Patronek GJ, Glickman LT (2003) Benefits of prophylactic gastropexy for dogs at risk of gastric dilatation-volvulus. *Prev. Vet. Med.* **60**(4): 319–29.

17.6   Further reading

Hulley SB, Cummings SR, Browner WS, Grady DG, Newman TB (2007) Utilizing Existing Databases. In: *Designing Clinical Research*, 3rd edn, Lippincott Williams and Wilkins, Philadelphia, pp 207–244.

17.7   MCQs

1 *Decision trees are composed of:*

(a)   decision nodes
(b)   chance nodes
(c)   terminal nodes
(d)   all of these.

2 *Decision tree decision nodes are nodes where:*

(a)   a conscious decision between two or more options is made
(b)   no decisions are made but likelihoods are attached to each outcome derived from the chance node, and the likelihoods or

probabilities of the outcomes emanating from a chance node add up to 1.0 or 100% respectively

(c) utilities are attached to these nodes to indicate the value attached to the outcome by the owner.

3 *Decision tree chance nodes are nodes where:*

(a) a conscious decision between two or more options is made

(b) no decisions are made but likelihoods are attached to each outcome derived from the chance node, and the likelihoods or probabilities of the outcomes emanating from a chance node add up to 1.0 or 100% respectively

(c) utilities are attached to these nodes to indicate the value attached to the outcome by the owner.

4 *Decision tree terminal nodes are nodes where:*

(a) a conscious decision between two or more options is made

(b) no decisions are made but likelihoods are attached to each outcome derived from the chance node, and the likelihoods or probabilities of the outcomes emanating from a chance node add up to 1.0 or 100% respectively

(c) utilities are attached to these nodes to indicate the value attached to the outcome by the owner.

5 *Owner utilities can be obtained by using:*

(a) dialogue
(b) visual analogue scales
(c) time trade-off calculations
(d) standard gamble techniques
(e) all of the above.

6 *When calculating treatment and testing thresholds possible outcomes may be:*

(a) probability of disease in the patient is below the testing threshold
(b) probability of disease in the patient is between the testing and treating threshold (the testing band)

(c) probability of disease in the patient is above the treating threshold
(d) (a) and (b) and (c)
(e) none of the above.

7 *Which of the following statements about case reports is false?*

(a) A case report is usually about a rare condition.
(b) A case report usually describes the clinical signs of a condition.
(c) A case report provides strong evidence for the cause of a condition.
(d) Case reports may give atypical descriptions.
(e) Case reports are useful as an early warning system of new and emerging diseases.

8 *Critically appraised topics:*

(a) are unpublished reviews of the literature
(b) are available on websites
(c) can be peer reviewed
(d) provide the answers to focused clinical questions
(e) are all of the above.

9 *Meta-analysis is:*

(a) a statistical analysis of the combined data of more than one study with similar experimental designs
(b) a technique to combine data from different experimental designs
(c) a literature review of literature reviews
(d) a statistical analysis of all the studies on a topic
(e) all of the above.

10 *A systematic review:*

(a) is likely to provide the strongest evidence
(b) may include a meta-analysis
(c) uses inclusion and exclusion criteria
(d) grades the quality of the studies
(e) is all of the above.

17.8 MCQ answers

1. (d); 2. (a); 3. (b); 4. (c); 5. (e); 6. (d); 7. (c); 8. (e); 9. (a); 10. (e)

INDEX

DATE DUE

APR 1 6			

GAYLORD   PRINTED IN U.S.A.